Cancer Metastasis and Cancer Stem Cell/Niche

Edited by:

Takanori Kawaguchi

Division of Human Life Sciences
Fukushima Medical University School of Nursing
Fukushima
Japan
&
Department of Pathology
General Aizu Chuo Hospital
Fukushima
Japan

Cancer Metastasis and Cancer Stem Cell/Niche

Editor: Takanori Kawaguchi

ISBN (eBook): 978-1-68108-347-6

ISBN (Print): 978-1-68108-348-3

First published in 2016.

Acknowledgements

I make a grateful acknowledgement for Mrs. Michiko Hoshi, who works in preparation of this book.

advertisements or ideas contained in the Work.

Limitation of Liability:

In no event will Bentham Science Publishers, its staff, editors and/or authors, be liable for any damages, including, without limitation, special, incidental and/or consequential damages and/or damages for lost data and/or profits arising out of (whether directly or indirectly) the use or inability to use the Work. The entire liability of Bentham Science Publishers shall be limited to the amount actually paid by you for the Work.

General:

1. Any dispute or claim arising out of or in connection with this License Agreement or the Work (including non-contractual disputes or claims) will be governed by and construed in accordance with the laws of the U.A.E. as applied in the Emirate of Dubai. Each party agrees that the courts of the Emirate of Dubai shall have exclusive jurisdiction to settle any dispute or claim arising out of or in connection with this License Agreement or the Work (including non-contractual disputes or claims).

2. Your rights under this License Agreement will automatically terminate without notice and without the need for a court order if at any point you breach any terms of this License Agreement. In no event will any delay or failure by Bentham Science Publishers in enforcing your compliance with this License Agreement constitute a waiver of any of its rights.

3. You acknowledge that you have read this License Agreement, and agree to be bound by its terms and conditions. To the extent that any other terms and conditions presented on any website of Bentham Science Publishers conflict with, or are inconsistent with, the terms and conditions set out in this License Agreement, you acknowledge that the terms and conditions set out in this License Agreement shall prevail.

Bentham Science Publishers Ltd.
Executive Suite Y - 2
PO Box 7917, Saif Zone
Sharjah, U.A.E.
Email: subscriptions@benthamscience.org

BENTHAM SCIENCE

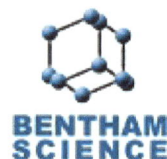

CONTENTS

FOREWORD

Our knowledge of cancer progression has grown exponentially since the discovery of oncogenes and our ability to model carcinogenesis and cancer initiation. Still the major challenge faced by physicians is the prevention and treatment of metastasis, the main reason for cancer related deaths. Our understanding of metastasis has lagged behind that of primary tumor biology and even with a surge in metastasis research we are far behind grasping its complexities.

Progress has been hampered by the research paradigm itself, which states that metastasis is an extremely late event in micro-evolutionary and temporal scales and driven by a tumor centric view. This information was mostly derived from models that use highly genetically aberrant and aggressive cancer cell line models and ignored the tumor microenvironment in the target organs. Thus, the field has accepted that metastases are an aggressive variant of the primary tumor and that these lesions share most characteristics that are mostly autonomous. This conclusion supported that primary tumor information should be sufficient to target the metastasis. So far this paradigm has shown moderate success at best in revealing the intricacies of metastasis and very little in yielding successful therapies to stop metastasis.

This book on metastasis is timely as we are at a turning point in metastasis research, which will impact the future of patient's treatment. The focus of this book is key to highlight how little we understand about cancer metastasis but also shows how great progress has been made in understanding the complexities of metastasis. This includes accepting that the complexities of metastasis biology are different from the primary tumor and that the target organ microenvironments play key roles in defining the biology of the metastatic cancer cells.

The chapters in this book are centered around the idea that there are minor populations in primary tumors termed cancer stem cells or cancer initiating cells that appear to also have the power to fuel metastasis. The chapters cover the role of the microenvironment composed by stromal cells and immune cells in determining the fate of the primary tumor and metastasis progression. The role of pre-metastatic microenvironments is also highlighted and the cancer stem cell concept is integrated with how niche signals impact epigenetic mechanisms that affect the expression of surface markers such as glycans to regulate the CSC behavior. The authors also cover the areas of secreted vesicles as important signaling mediators between the tumor and the stroma and the role of angiogenesis, which is a clear factor for metastatic maintenances. One chapter is focused on the development of imaging modalities to improve the detection of rare cell subpopulations in tumor lesions, and such advancements are critically needed. This becomes critical when thinking that after surgery and treatment and before metastatic outgrowth there is a period of minimal residual disease (MRD). This periods can last for decades when the seeds of metastasis are dormant and for which we have no evidence-based treatment and imaging modalities. Unfortunately this stems primarily from the lack of our understanding of the biology that defines MRD, dormancy and reactivation. However, the chapters will illustrate that the field has moved forward significantly and new findings are routinely published that are expanding our understanding of metastasis and how to target it.

As mentioned before this book comes at a time when a change is needed if we are going to be successful in targeting metastasis and that requires deepening our understanding of the biology of disseminated disease, developing markers to detect it, image it and come up with new therapeutic strategies that are based on the direct knowledge of MRD biology and metastasis and not inferred from extrapolations based on primary tumor information, that is sometimes gathered a decade or more before manifestation of the metastasis and thus may be a very different disease. The work highlighted in this book is a testament of the excellent work being developed worldwide to target this deadly step of the disease and possibly our best short-term chance to change the course of cancer treatment and improve patient's life.

Julio Aguirre-Ghiso
Division of Hematology and Oncology
Department of Medicine
Department of Otolaryngology
Department of Oncological Sciences
Tisch Cancer Institute at Mount Sinai
Ichan School of Medicine at Mount Sinai
New York, USA

PREFACE

A malignant tumor is an actively growing tissue, composed of cells derived from a single cell that has undergone abnormal irreversible differentiation. These cells have two fundamental qualities: invasion and metastasis that induce the risk of cancer. Interestingly, recent researchers suggest that a malignant tumor is originated from cancer stem cells (CSC) accompanied with the niches. In this eBook, I would like to ask how the invasion and metastasis of cancer cells are explained by CSC theory and/or niche theory. The major points are as follows.

1. The fundamental aspects of cancer:
   1. The first point of discussion is about the CSC/ niche in carcinoma *in situ* lesion which appears in various types of cancer including breast and bladder cancers. Where is the niche corresponding to CSC in the above situation and what is the role of the niche in cancer progression?
   2. Cancer metastasis involves two characteristic occurrences: "organ preference metastasis" and "metastatic potential". Can these metastatic characteristics be explained by CSC /niche theory well?
2. Metastatic phenotypes:
   The mechanisms of cancer metastasis include non-invasiveness (carcinoma *in situ*), lateral/side invasion, stromal invasion, intravasation, circulation, arrest, attachment, extravasation, early growth, growth, and sometimes secondary/tertiary metastasis. This is followed by cellular/molecular mechanisms including cellular adhesion molecules such as carbohydrates, chemotactic activity by producing pseudopodia and invadopodia, deformability/plasticity and cytostreaming of metastatic cancer cells, and survival of metastatic cancer cells in floating (substrate-independent condition). Can these phenotypes of metastatic cancer cells be explained by cancer stem cell theory?
3. The goal of this study is clinical application of the knowledge obtained by CSC/niche theory. CSC/niche targets have important therapeutic implications. The role of CSC/ niche on therapies for the prevention, maintenance therapy, personalized care, and perhaps even integrative care of cancer will be discussed.

Takanori Kawaguchi
Division of Human Life Sciences
Fukushima Medical University School of Nursing, Fukushima, Japan
Department of Pathology
General Aizu Chuo Hospital, Fukushima, Japan

Biography

My research on cancer metastasis began in 1968, at the 2nd Department of Pathology, Fukushima Medical University College of Medicine (Professor and Chairman, Kyuya Nakamura) and continued till 2006. Since 2006, I have been working at the Division of Nursing (Professor and Chairman, Takashi Honda) and the Department of Pathology, Aizu Chuo Hospital (Head, Takanori Kawaguchi). During this period, I collaborated with many researchers. In 1980, I visited the Department of Tumor Biology, MD Anderson Cancer Center and Tumor Institute in Houston (Professor and Chairman, Garth L. Nicolson), where I studied the metastasis of B16 melanoma variant sublines for a year. During the past 50 years, there have been great advances in metastasis research, for example, electron microscopy revealed cellular/subcellular behavior of tumor cells in metastasis. Molecular biology facilitated identification of the molecules involved in metastasis. For the last 100 years, the biggest issue associated with cancer metastasis research was a conflict of "anatomical-mechanical theory" and "seed and soil theory." However, our research indicated that the anatomical–mechanical theory can be replaced by tissue injury hypothesis (microinjury hypothesis), and this concept was supported by the large scale of research on human cancer. Thus, I believe that metastasis occurs in the affinity of tumor cells and soil (niche), where soil causes the tumor cells to become immature.

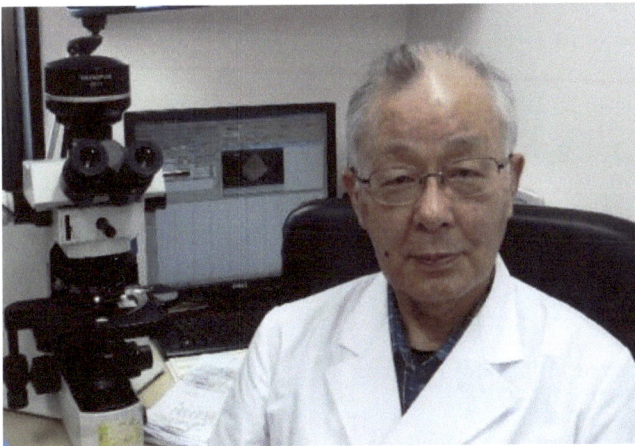

Takanori Kawaguchi

List of Contributors

Atsuko Deguchi	Department of Pharmacology, Tokyo Women's Medical University, Tokyo, Japan
Bi-He Cai	The Institute of Biomedical Sciences (IBMS), Academia Sinica, Taipei, Taiwan
Danny R. Welch	Department of Cancer Biology, The University of Kansas Medical Center, Kansas, USA Department of Pathology and Laboratory Medicine, University of Kansas Medical Center, Kansas, USA The University of Kansas Cancer Center, Kansas, USA
Dorcas A. Annan	Vascular Biology, Frontier Research Unit, Institute for Genetic Medicine, Hokkaido University, Sapporo, Japan
Eric D. Young	Department of Cancer Biology, The University of Kansas Medical Center, Kansas, USA
Fariba Behbod	Department of Cancer Biology, The University of Kansas Medical Center, Kansas, USA Department of Pathology and Laboratory Medicine, University of Kansas Medical Center, Kansas, USA The University of Kansas Cancer Center, Kansas, USA
Hsiang-Chi Huang	The Institute of Biomedical Sciences (IBMS), Academia Sinica, Taipei, Taiwan
Keiichiro Sakuma	Division of Molecular Pathology, Aichi Cancer Center, Nagoya, Japan
Koji Morimoto	Department of Hepato-Biliary-Pancreatic Surgery, Osaka National Hospital, Osaka, Japan Osaka Women's Junior College, Osaka, Japan
Kyoko Hida	Vascular Biology, Frontier Research Unit, Institute for Genetic Medicine, Hokkaido University, Sapporo, Japan
Linheng Li	Department of Cancer Biology, The University of Kansas Medical Center, Kansas, USA Stowers Institute for Medical Research (SIMR), Missouri, USA The University of Kansas Cancer Center, Kansas, USA
Nako Maishi	Vascular Biology, Frontier Research Unit, Institute for Genetic Medicine, Hokkaido University, Sapporo, Japan
Reiji Kannagi	The Institute of Biomedical Sciences (IBMS), Academia Sinica, Taipei, Taiwan Advanced Medical Research Center, Aichi Medical University, Nagakute, Japan
Shoji Nakamori	Department of Hepato-Biliary-Pancreatic Surgery, Osaka National Hospital, Osaka, Japan
Takeshi Tomita	Department of Pharmacology, Tokyo Women's Medical University, Tokyo, Japan

Yasuhiro Hida   Department of Cardiovascular and Thoracic Surgery, Hokkaido University Graduate School of Medicine, Sapporo, Japan

Yoshiro Maru   Department of Pharmacology, Tokyo Women's Medical University, Tokyo, Japan

Fundamental Relationships Between Cancer Stem Cells, the Cancer Stem Cell Niche and Metastasis

Eric D. Young[1]**, Linheng Li**[1,2,4]**, Fariba Behbod**[1,3,4] **and Danny R. Welch**[1,3,4,*]

[1] *Department of Cancer Biology, The University of Kansas Medical Center, Kansas, USA*

[2] *Stowers Institute for Medical Research (SIMR), Missouri, USA*

[3] *Department of Pathology and Laboratory Medicine, University of Kansas Medical Center, Kansas, USA*

[4] *The University of Kansas Cancer Center, Kansas, USA*

Abstract: Parallels drawn between stem cells and cancer are not new. However, these shared features are becoming increasingly important as our understanding of disseminated, recurrent and metastatic cancer cell biology continues to develop. Indeed, nearly all cancer-related deaths are the result of recurrent and metastatic disease, highlighting the need for a more comprehensive schema of how tumors colonize new sites, resist therapy and evolve. In this chapter, we compare the phenotypes of stem cells, cancer stem cells (CSCs) and metastatic cells, highlighting notable points of contrast. We begin with an introduction to stem cell biology, tumor-initiating CSCs, metastatic cells and discuss shared features. The implication of the stem-like phenotype extends to many characteristics of cell biology: cell division, differentiation, morphology, gene expression, motility, invasion, clonogenicity, capacity for colonization, metabolism and the interaction of these cells with their surrounding microenvironment. Stem cell phenotypes are highly complex and, while there may be a number of shared features, there are important elements that are uniquely tissue-dependent. While staunch definitions based upon a single biomarker of stemness have proven inadequate in broader applications, seeing universal themes of the stem cell phenotype will provide critical insights for studying cancer. Our understanding of this complex biology is critical for developing rational and dynamic therapeutic interventions for patients with recurrent and metastatic cancer.

* Corresponding author Danny R. Welch: Department of Cancer Biology, The University of Kansas Medical Center, 3901 Rainbow Blvd., Wahl Hall West 2003, Mailstop 1071, Kansas City, Kansas, 66160, USA; Tel: +1-913-945-7739; Fax: +1-913-588-4701; Email: dwelch@kumc.edu.

Takanori Kawaguchi (Ed.)

Keywords: Biomarker, Cancer stem cell, Cancer stem cell niche, Clonogenicity, Dissemination, Dormancy, Epithelial-mesenchymal transition, Heterogeneity, Metabolism, Metastasis, Metastasis-initiating cells, Metastatic cell, Metastatic colonization, Metastatic niche, Pluripotency, Quiescence, Review, Self-renewal, Stem cell, Stem cell niche, Tumor progression, Tumorigenesis, Tumorigenic cells, Tumor-initiating cell.

INTRODUCTION

The observation that features of a cancer cell resemble developmentally primitive cells dates back over 150 years [1]. This has proven to be a perspicacious observation indeed, given the similarities between cancer cells and stem cells with respect to their dynamic regulation of mitosis, gene expression, migration, metabolism and self-sustainability. Cell division is a critical component of carcinogenesis and early observations prompted the notion that cancer may arise from a stem cell [2, 3]. Additionally, the therapeutic significance of cancer cells displaying a stem cell-like phenotype has been more recently appreciated after patients whose cancer was treated with chemotherapy and were without evidence of disease, experienced recurrence of disease months or years later. These observations suggested that there was perhaps a population of mitotically quiescent cancer cells unaffected by chemotherapy that survived, proliferated and gave rise to the recurrent tumor or metastatic disease [4]. Tumor-initiating cells are the proposed "cancer stem cells" (CSCs). Given the importance of these phenotypes in the control of cancer, here we compare the shared and distinct biological features of normal stem cells, CSCs and metastatic cancer cells and consider the therapeutic significance of these insights.

FEATURES OF STEMNESS

Stem Cells in Normal Physiology and Development

Stem cells are populations of cells with the capacity to divide symmetrically, where the resulting daughter cells retain an equal potential to produce cells of a given lineage, or asymmetrically, resulting in more differentiated daughter cells that are narrowed in the variety of cells in that lineage they can produce [5]. *In vivo,* it was thought that stem cells spend the majority of their cell cycle in mitotic quiescence [6], and upon stimulation by tissue damage or exogenous factors they can be induced to divide. More recently, in addition to quiescent stem cells, it has been shown that a population of Lgr5$^+$stem cells also undergo active proliferation [7]. Daughter cells resulting from asymmetric divisions may become the more actively proliferating yet shorter-lived transit-amplifying cells which serve to regenerate tissue when required [8]. When stem cells are cultured *in vitro* however, conventional passaging methods may select for rapidly proliferating cells [9], explaining in part the dissonance between these two phenotypes. Ultimately, the orchestrated proliferation and differentiation of normal stem cells serve to reconstitute tissue lost to damage, aging and use. In a similar way, tumor cells remaining after selection by chemotherapy would be the "stem cells" of that tumor. These CSCs could eventually be stimulated to divide, resulting in the maintenance of slow-cycling CSCs. Stochastic changes in other daughter cells would re-establish tumor heterogeneity and a population of rapidly dividing cancer cells responsible for recurrence of disease.

The Cancer Stem Cell Phenotype

Morphology, Differentiation and Self Renewal

Discussion of CSCs envelops many concepts related to the origin of malignant cells, how selective processes change the tumor cell population over time (*i.e.* tumor progression), the ability of cells to successfully colonize new sites (*i.e.* metastasis), and the features of therapy-resistant cancer cells in disease recurrence (summarized in Table **1** and Fig. **1**). Although a so-called "tumor initiating cell" may very well fit many of the aforementioned criteria, this nomenclature describes many of the later aspects of CSC biology without reference necessarily to their origin, with which we begin our discussion. Morphologic observations of cancers and embryonic tissues gave rise to the first ideas connecting cancer with stem cells. The strikingly heterogeneous composition of teratomas, containing teeth, hair, and sundry embryonic tissues led to the hypothesis that these tumors may come from a stem cell [10]. Further studies extended this observation and demonstrated the stemness of teratoma cells by showing their potential to differentiate into a multitude of tissues [11]. Beyond potency, normal stem cells, tumorigenic cancer cells and metastatic cells must all have the capacity for continued proliferation, from even a single cell [12]. However, it was observed in leukemia that many of the cancer cells had a finite ability to self-renew, which incited the search for the tumor-sustaining CSCs in this disease. Cell surface markers were used to define a subpopulation of human $CD34^+CD38^-$ acute myeloid leukemia (AML) cells capable of recapitulating an AML phenotype in SCID mice [13]. This subpopulation was less differentiated than the other cells and provided evidence that a defined population of resident stem cells is responsible for AML.

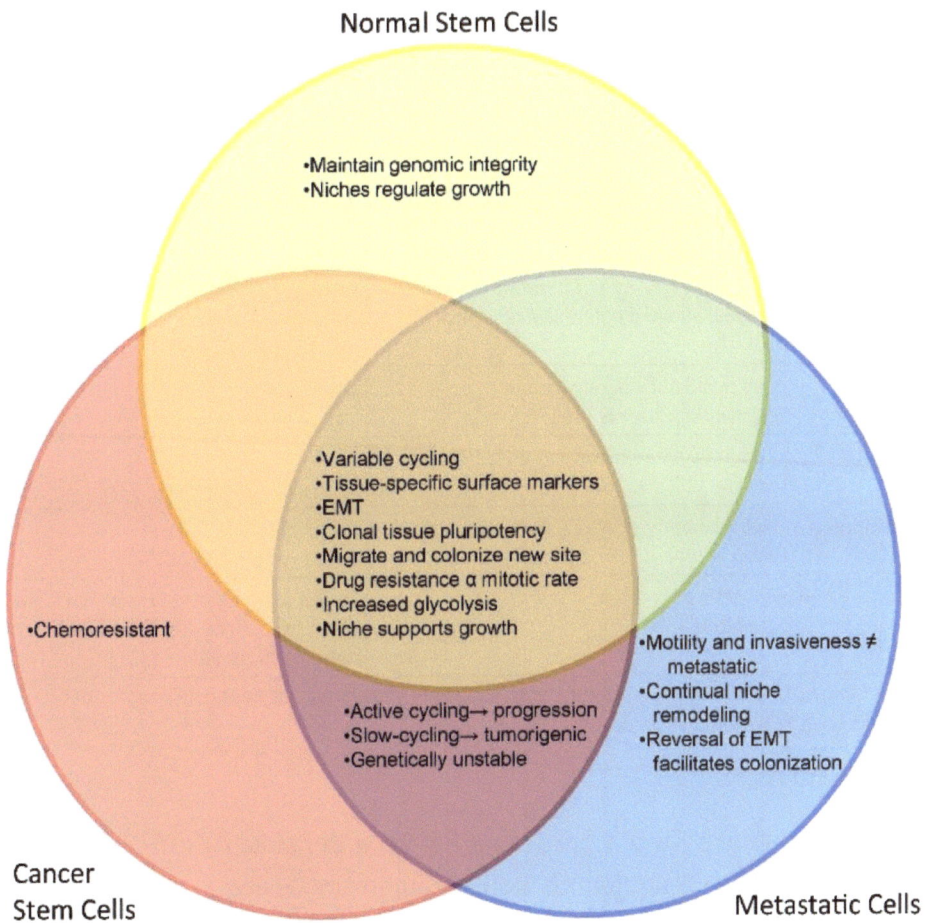

Normal Stem Cells

•Maintain genomic integrity
•Niches regulate growth

•Variable cycling
•Tissue-specific surface markers
•EMT
•Clonal tissue pluripotency
•Migrate and colonize new site
•Drug resistance α mitotic rate
•Increased glycolysis
•Niche supports growth

•Chemoresistant

•Motility and invasiveness ≠ metastatic
•Continual niche remodeling
•Reversal of EMT facilitates colonization

•Active cycling→ progression
•Slow-cycling→ tumorigenic
•Genetically unstable

Cancer
Stem Cells

Metastatic Cells

Fig. (1). Properties of stem cells, cancer stem cells and metastatic cells.

Table 1. Similarities between stem cells, cancer stem cells and metastatic cells*.

	Shared Features	Distinguishing Features
Mitotic Rate	Both slow and actively-cycling populations exist [6, 14].	Slow-cycling CSC populations are tumorigenic and can be chemotherapy resistant [17]. Actively-cycling CSC populations drive tumor progression [18].
Genomic Integrity	Normal stem cells maintain their genomic integrity.	CSCs [74] and metastatic cells [75] are genetically unstable.
Dormancy/ Quiescence	Cells may remain dormant or be triggered to actively proliferate [6].	
Surface Markers	Common markers are shared in mammary cells [30] and hematopoietic stem cell [13].	Stem cell, CSC and metastatic cells markers vary by tissue. Markers may also vary within a tissue [23 - 25].
EMT	Expression of EMT related markers can be observed [30, 45, 61].	Reversal of EMT (MET) related markers facilitates metastatic colonization [44, 57].
Self-Renewal	Must be able to self-sustain and reconstitute the tissue, even from a single clone [8, 13].	
Motility	Have the capacity to migrate from the original site and colonize a new site [29, 46].	Motility may or may not correlate with metastatic capacity [29, 40].
Invasiveness	Can invade or migrate through surrounding tissues [46, 76]	Invasiveness is necessary but not sufficient for metastasis [43, 76].
Metabolism	Generally show increased glycolytic activity [29, 33, 36, 53].	
Drug Resistance	Not inherently drug resistant, depends upon mitotic rate and phenotype [25, 28].	Drug resistance does not guarantee metastatic potential [25, 28, 38].
Niche	Provides protection, support and regulates growth [63, 66].	Cancer associated niches do not suppress respective cells. Metastatic niches are continually remodeled [77].

*: While not exhaustive, this table highlights general trends and shared features between normal stem cells, cancer stem cells (CSCs) and metastatic cells.

Mitotic Activity

There is also evidence for a relationship between the state of differentiation and tumorigenic capacity in squamous cell carcinomas, where it was demonstrated that poorly differentiated cells were the fastest cycling cells in the tumor [14]. As squamous cell carcinoma cancer cells differentiated they became less mitotically active and less tumorigenic, suggesting that there was a primordial population of cells responsible for persistence of the tumor and that the cancer cells entered mitotic quiescence as they differentiated. The net mitotic index of malignant cancer cells is generally constitutively high, a feature that has been exploited by conventional chemotherapies for the past 75 years [15]. Stem cells in the hilum of the ovary have been demonstrated to be both slow-cycling and prone to tumorigenesis after tumor-suppressor loss [16], suggesting a role for these slow-cycling, normal stem cells in the development of ovarian carcinomas. CSCs are hypothesized to have a low mitotic rate that aids in rendering them resistant to traditional chemotherapeutics targeting rapidly proliferating cells. Supporting this hypothesis, a relatively slow-cycling population of CSCs was shown to drive tumor growth in glioblastoma [17]. In an intestinal adenoma model, it was demonstrated that Lgr5[+] stem cells divide and contribute to tumorigenesis, although this cycling population was unable to reinitiate tumors [18]. These results emphasize that a cycling subset of CSCs contribute to tumor progression, although they may be intrinsically sensitive to treatments targeting rapidly proliferating cells. Slower-cycling CSCs are important in tumorigenesis and in driving recurrence of disease, especially in the context of a post-chemotherapeutic setting.

Protein and Biomarker Expression

While these data suggest that tumor initiating cells have the capacity for continued proliferation and differentiation, the identity of CSCs in many solid tumors remains unclear. Solid tumors are a complex amalgamation of normal (endothelial cells, fibroblasts, immune cells, *etc.*) and neoplastic cells whose dynamic interaction may positively [19, 20] or negatively regulate tumor progression [21] and metastasis [22]. In the absence of morphologic features to distinguish differentiated cancer cells from stem cells, biomarkers of these states are required. Identifying appropriate biomarkers and physically separating them from their surrounding microenvironment makes the lineage tracing and clonal passaging experiments required for definitive demonstration of CSC contributions in solid tumors challenging.

It is expected that markers of solid tumor CSCs will be unique to their tissue of origin (*i.e.* markers of breast CSCs will differ from intestinal CSCs) just as markers of normal stem cells vary by tissue, there are not yet unified markers of solid tumor CSCs within a given tissue, although many candidates have been identified. This is illustrated by data from mammary tumors, where a population of cells defined by CD44$^+$/CD24^{-low} expression was shown to have an increased capacity for tumorigenesis [23]. Other groups have identified CD61/β3 integrin as biologically relevant markers used to identify mammary CSCs [24]. Stem cell antigen 1 (Sca1) has also been identified as a marker of mammary stem cells, which are also resistant to ionizing radiation [25]. This variation in mammary stem cell markers could be a consequence of technical variation or differences in the model systems.

However, these data might also suggest that, in the mammary gland, the CSC phenotype may not be solely dependent upon a static, defined set of biomarkers. Instead, the tumorigenic and differentiating capacity of CSCs reflects a multitude of intrinsic and environmental factors. In this case, the expression of various biomarkers may be an effect and not a cause of more profound biological interactions. Indeed, in solid tumors a number of prospective biomarkers have been proposed [23, 26 - 30], but it is unlikely that a uniform set will concisely define CSC biology. As compared to carcinomas, tumors of neural crest origin may have different capacity for, and regulators of, tumorigenesis and metastasis [31]. Thus, while there may be unifying principles guiding the activity and significance of CSCs, the molecular means by which they arrive at these common ends are plastic.

Metabolism

Altered cell metabolism is another shared feature between stem cells, CSCs and metastatic cells. The propensity of cancer cells to use primarily aerobic glycolysis as opposed to oxidative phosphorylation (OXPHOS) has been known for almost 90 years [32] and has been observed in stem cells more recently [33 - 35]. Ovarian cancer cells grown in spheroid culture consumed higher amounts of glucose than their counterparts cultured in 2D culture, demonstrated expression of stem-cell related genes and had increased tumorigenic capacity [29]. In melanoma cells whose metabolism was comprised primarily of aerobic glycolysis readily metastasized, whereas those whose metabolism had been shifted toward OXPHOS did not [36].

Importantly, while both stem cells and cancer cells have increased glycolytic activity as compared to most differentiated and mitotically quiescent cells in the body, differences between the two would permit the targeting of cancer cells, while preserving normal stem cell function. Illustrating such a difference, hematopoietic stem cells (HSCs), hematopoietic progenitor cells and leukemia cells were sensitive to a reduction in lactate dehydrogenase (LDHA), but the HSCs could tolerate reduced levels of the upstream glycolytic enzyme pyruvate kinase (M2 isoform), whereas the hematopoietic progenitor cells and leukemia cells could not [37]. The authors propose that this gap between the metabolic requirements of HSCs and leukemic cells offers a therapeutically tractable window. These results draw an association between the metabolism of stem cells, CSCs, and metastatic cells suggesting that cell metabolism may be a powerful parameter for assessing or treating neoplastic disease.

Metastasis Initiating Cells

Critical Components of Metastasis

Metastatic cancer cells are defined by the ability to leave the primary tumor, enter and survive in the circulation, arrest and extravasate at a different site and proliferate at the secondary site to form a metastatic colony [38]. Enhancing any step along this cascade has the potential to increase metastatic efficacy, while a deficiency in any step will definitively avert metastasis. Far less than one percent of the cells that enter the circulation are capable of forming a metastatic colony [39] and if disseminated cells are prevented from outgrowth after arriving at the secondary site, they will not form a metastatic colony [40]. What then are the factors that are required for successful metastatic outgrowth?

Metastatic lesions are commonly associated with aggressive primary tumors with a high mitotic rate, although competition for resources within an actively proliferating tumor cannot solely explain the progression of metastatic disease. However, these trends are punctuated by numerous exceptions, concluding an imperfect relationship. For example, carcinoid tumors readily metastasize despite their generally indolent growth rates [41, 42]. In the skin, basal cell carcinomas, glioblastoma multiforme [38], and desmoid tumors [43] are readily invasive, yet rarely metastatic. Thus, an invasive tumor is not necessarily metastatic if these cells fail to colonize a new site. Mechanisms by which normal stem cells from the neural crest migrate to and colonize new tissues may share common biologic means with metastatic cells which are required to complete similar tasks to survive and proliferate to colonize new tissues.

Epithelial-to-Mesenchymal Transition

During development, cells leave the crest of the neural tube, migrate and become incorporated into tissues such as the facial bones, skin and gut. Their delamination from the neural tube, migration and accompanying phenotypic changes are known as the epithelial-to-mesenchymal transition (EMT). Similar changes are hypothesized to occur as epithelial cells from a carcinoma leave the primary tumor and migrate to a potential metastatic site. As the epithelial phenotype is also observed in metastatic cells, the reverse changes are thought to occur at the metastatic site, a process known as mesenchymal to epithelial transition (MET) [44]. Classically, the increased motility of cells having undergone EMT is facilitated by decrease in the cell adhesion protein E-cadherin and increases in the expression of the intermediate filament protein vimentin and the transcription factors Snail, Slug and Twist. Changes in similar gene expression patterns have been observed in metastasis [45], however to elicit changes in metastatic efficacy the functional consequences of these EMT-like changes must extend beyond facilitating cell delamination and migration.

Expression of the transcription factors Slug and Sox9 have been identified as markers of the basal and stem cells in the mammary epithelium [30]. Their expression increases the capacity of mammary epithelial cells to form organoids *in vitro* and reconstitute the mammary gland, suggesting that Slug and Sox9 are markers of the stem cells in the mammary epithelium. In addition, knockdown of Slug and Sox9 decreased formation of macroscopic metastases in an intravenous (IV) experimental metastasis model, correlating the stem cell phenotype with efficacy of metastatic colonization at the secondary site by disseminated cancer cells. During normal development, Sox9 functions to sustain migrating cells from the neural crest on their journey to the peripheral tissues [46]. Although Slug and Sox9 have been detected in human breast cancers, they have not been identified as markers in metastatic breast tumors per se [30].

There exist other normal physiologic processes that mirror activities of metastatic tumor cells. Hematopoietic cells and immune cells migrate to a distant site and extravasate in response to chemokines. The C-X-C chemokine receptor type 4 (CXCR4) and C-X-C motif chemokine 12 (CXCL12 or stromal-derived factor 1/SDF-1) receptor-ligand relationship functions in normal physiology to attract lymphocytes to sites of inflammation [47] or to the bone marrow [48], and is also overexpressed in cancer cells which metastasize to the bone [49]. Thus, genes that facilitate metastasis may reflect a commandeering of normal developmental and immune programs. Interestingly, expression of CXCR4 has been shown to be upregulated by transformation-related protein 63 (TP63), conferring increased capacity for colony formation, anchorage-independent growth and chemotaxis [50]. These results suggest that there is overlap between the features of metastatic cancer cells and stem cells, despite the fact that these data do not demonstrate direct evidence for increased capacity of CXCR4 expressing cells to colonize the secondary site and complete the metastatic cascade. Thus, in many cases, metastatic cells are co-opting normal processes and mechanisms to facilitate progression of disease.

Mechanisms of Metastasis

Intriguingly, the induction of EMT results in not only expression of the expected mesenchymal proteins, but also of markers of stem cells [51]. These mammary cells were also more tumorigenic after having undergone EMT. Expression of Twist was shown to be required for metastasis of mammary carcinoma cells [52]. In pancreatic cancer, expression of Snail maintained expression of aldehyde dehydrogenase (ALDH), considered to be a marker of stem cells [53]. Hypoxia can induce EMT [54] and other pro-survival pathways. Subsequent up-regulation of HIF-1α and related target genes is a mechanism by which cells increase motility, invasiveness and their capacity to cope with increased amounts of unfolded proteins, serving to enhance metastasis [55].

However in colon cancer driven by L1, a neural cell adhesion molecule downstream of β-Catenin, changes in EMT related genes were not observed in cells overexpressing L1. These cells demonstrated increased motility, invasiveness and capacity for metastasis (L1-mediated colon cancer cell metastasis does not require changes in EMT and cancer stem cell markers). Others would suggest that the changes observed within EMT are within the plasticity of epithelial function, and that the changes observed do not necessarily provide evidence for differences in cell identity [56]. These results suggest that metastasis and the factors facilitating metastatic colonization do not necessarily require EMT, although EMT-like changes in gene expression are one means by which to arrive at the same biological end.

Disseminated cancer cells must arrest, survive and proliferate at the secondary site to form a metastatic colony. Interestingly, suppression of EMT related genes appear to indeed be one component of successful colonization. Loss of the homeobox gene Prrx1 both abolished the EMT phenotype and was shown to be required for successful metastatic colonization [57]. An epigenetic regulator of homeobox genes, Bmi-1, was shown to direct self-renewal in mammary cells [58] and has also been shown to be required for tumorigenesis in colon cancer [59]. However, overexpression of the homeobox gene Goosecoid was found to increase both the motility of breast cancer cells *in vitro* and the number of metastases in an experimental metastasis model [60]. The observation that both overexpression of homeobox genes (Goosecoid) and suppression of homeobox genes (Prrx1) result in increased metastasis suggest that there remains much to be understood about the temporal and spatial regulation of EMT-related genes with respect to their influence on metastatic efficacy. Doublecortin-like kinase 1 DCLK1, found in circulating CSCs [61] and overexpressed in renal cell carcinoma, was found to regulate EMT in these cells and to have a distinct pattern of promoter methylation [62]. These data suggest that epigenetic regulation may be a common mechanism regulating the activity of normal stem cells, CSCs and metastatic cells that govern cell decisions regarding renewal and differentiation.

Contributions of the Niche

The Normal Stem Cell Niche

The architecture of the stem cell niche is tissue dependent, but in all cases it refers to the three-dimensional space surrounding normal stem cells that provides the stem cells with physical protection, nutrients and signals that direct stem cell behavior [63]. Indeed, one of the functions of the stem cell niche is to regulate the proliferation of stem cells to ensure that these cells with such profound proliferative capacity do not divide continuously [64]. Thus, the absence of the stem cell niche *in vitro* to suppress unnecessary proliferation also helps to explain the brisk mitotic phenotype observed there, in addition to any added effect the process of conventional cell culture may contribute toward selecting for rapidly dividing cells.

The CSC Niche

The niche supporting CSCs by definition then differs in this regard [65], as proliferating cancer cells have already overridden growth inhibitory signals. Like the niche of the normal stem cell, the CSC niche provides the requisite protection and nutrients for CSCs [66] and indeed may use the same signaling molecules to influence the mitotic activity of CSCs [67]. The importance of maintaining dormancy is also highlighted in the context of metastasis. Progression of metastatic disease may occur months to years after anticancer therapy, suggesting that disseminated cells existed in a dormant niche or state. What are the stimuli that induce this awakening from dormancy and what are the signals that would maintain it? Notch signaling was shown to regulate the proliferation and capacity for sphere formation of tumor cells in glioblastoma multiforme (GBM) [68]. The authors conclude from these data that Notch signaling promotes the CSC phenotype in GBM, although an alternative explanation might be that the GBM cells are dependent upon the endothelial cells and that the decrease in GBM CSC is an effect of a decrease in endothelial cell number.

The Metastatic Niche

By comparison, the metastatic niche refers to the immediate microenvironment surrounding disseminated and seeded, ostensibly metastatic cells and it also helps to facilitate cancer cell growth. The secondary site where disseminated cancer cells will eventually invade and proliferate as a metastatic colony is termed pre-metastatic niche before the arrival of the tumor cells [69]. Interestingly, the pre-metastatic niche has been shown to be "primed" by HSCs from the bone marrow prior to colonization by disseminated tumor cells [70]. This action is initiated by factors released from the primary tumor and results in upregulation of fibronectin in the niche fibroblasts and increased retention and growth of metastatic cells at the secondary site. Interestingly, the features of the normal stem cell niche may also provide necessary interactions to foster the growth of metastatic cells to those sites. For example, breast cancer cells metastatic to the bone received growth signals initiated by heterotypic cadherin interactions between the metastatic cells and the cells forming the osteoblastic and HSC niche [71]. The metastatic niche not only supports the growth of metastatic cancer cells, but is also dynamically regulated as the cells colonize the secondary site. Exosomes are one means by which this remodeling of the metastatic niche is mediated [72].

CONCLUSION

In conclusion, normal stem cells, CSCs and metastatic cells share many features including the ability to migrate [31, 46], synergistically interact with the surrounding microenvironment or niche for growth signals [19, 64, 70], resist apoptosis [5] and recapitulate from clonal origins the heterogeneity observed within the original tumor or tissue [13, 30]. The ability to successfully adapt to a changing environment is a necessary and shared feature of normal stem cells, CSCs and metastatic cells. Migratory stem cells of the neural crest and metastatic cancer cells must adapt to the physical environment at new locations while CSCs must adapt to changes in the local environment due to selective pressures present within a tumor (*e.g.* competition for nutrients or oxygen, anti-cancer therapy, *etc.*). One means by which this phenotypic plasticity is accomplished both during development and in cancer progression is by epigenetic regulation of gene expression. Dysregulation of the epigenome has already become a therapeutic target for cancer [73].

Requirements of a CSC include the ability to self-renew and proliferate indefinitely, to differentiate into cancer cells with more limited replicative potential and to be capable of reconstituting a tumor upon transfer. In essence, the fulfillment of Koch's postulates for CSCs of each tumor type will definitively establish the identity of the CSCs in various tumor types. However, isolation and serial passaging experiments required to definitively identify and study ostensible CSCs remain technically challenging, especially in solid tumors. For this reason, data by which groups provide evidence for CSC contribution in their tumor of interest vary greatly. As the identity of both CSCs and metastatic initiating cells continues to be elucidated, future therapeutic interventions must not rely upon a single biomarker for targeting and tumor destruction. Rather, a multi-faceted approach utilizing multiple, concurrent therapeutic interventions addressing different aspects of CSC biology is likely to be required for eradication of tumorigenic cancer cells. The reverse may also be true, as discoveries concerning CSCs and metastatic cells may also serve as a model for understanding the biology and regulation of normal stem cells, with important human applications for regenerative medicine. These considerations highlight significant remaining questions Table **2** regarding the *in vivo* biology of cancer sustaining cells and implications for treating patients with cancer.

Table 2. Remaining unanswered questions.

• What is the *in vivo* mitotic rate of cancer stem cells and metastatic cells?
• What triggers the awakening from dormancy of cancer stem cells that causes recurrence?
• What makes CSC and metastatic cancer cells genetically unstable?
• Why is the genetic instability from CSCs and metastatic cancer cells not self-limiting?
• What therapeutically targetable features distinguish CSCs from normal resident stem cells and other cells within the tumor?
• What traceable biomarkers can be used to detect CSCs?
• How will knowledge of CSCs direct patient treatment and follow-up?

As our understanding of the biology and the selective process that produces the CSCs and metastatic cells expands, we may begin to therapeutically intercede on multiple fronts. What matters most to patients in distinguishing normal stem cells, CSCs and metastatic cancer cells is the identification of therapeutically targetable features. Ultimately, the relevance of our understanding this biology will be determined by the degree to which improved treatments produce better outcomes for patients with recurrent, disseminated and metastatic cancer.

CONFLICT OF INTEREST

The authors confirm that they have no conflict of interest to declare for this publication.

ACKNOWLEDGEMENTS

Work from the Welch lab has been generously supported by grants from the National Foundation for Cancer Research (CA62168, CA87728, CA134981), National Foundation for Cancer Research Center for Metastasis Research, U.S. Army Medical Research Defense Command (DAMD-17-96-1-6152, DAMD17-02-1-0541, W81XWH-07-1-0540d), Susan G. Komen for the Cure (SAC110037), Kansas Biosciences Authority, Steiner Fund for Metastasis Research, Melanoma Research Foundation and METAvivor Inc. DRW is the Hall Family Professor of Molecular Medicine and is a Kansas Bioscience Authority Eminent Scholar.

REFERENCES

[1]   Virchow R. Editorial archive fur pathologische anatomie und physiologie fuer klinische medizin 1855; 23-54.

[2]   Durante F. Nesso fisio-patologico tra la struttura dei nei materni e la gentsi di alcuni tumori maligni. Arch Memor Observ Chir Prat 11 1874.

[3]   Cohnheim J. Congenitales, quergestreiftes muskelsarkon der nireren. Virchows Arch 1875; 65: 64. [http://dx.doi.org/10.1007/BF01978936]

[4]   Osella-Abate S, *et al.* Risk factors related to late metastases in 1,372 melanoma patients disease free more than 10 years. Int J Cancer 2014; 136(10): 2453-7.

[5]   Viatour P, Somervaille TC, Venkatasubrahmanyam S, *et al.* Hematopoietic stem cell quiescence is maintained by compound contributions of the retinoblastoma gene family. Cell Stem Cell 2008; 3(4): 416-28. [http://dx.doi.org/10.1016/j.stem.2008.07.009] [PMID: 18940733]

[6]   Cotsarelis G, Sun TT, Lavker RM. Label-retaining cells reside in the bulge area of pilosebaceous unit: implications for follicular stem cells, hair cycle, and skin carcinogenesis. Cell 1990; 61(7): 1329-37. [http://dx.doi.org/10.1016/0092-8674(90)90696-C] [PMID: 2364430]

[7]   Li L, Clevers H. Coexistence of quiescent and active adult stem cells in mammals. Science 2010; 327(5965): 542-5. [http://dx.doi.org/10.1126/science.1180794] [PMID: 20110496]

[8]   Necas E, Neuwirt J. Effect of hydroxyurea and vinblastine on the proliferation of the pluripotential stem cells. Neoplasma 1977; 24(1): 29-40. [PMID: 840337]

[9]   Richichi C, Brescia P, Alberizzi V, Fornasari L, Pelicci G. Marker-independent method for isolating slow-dividing cancer stem cells in human glioblastoma. Neoplasia 2013; 15(7): 840-7. [http://dx.doi.org/10.1593/neo.13662] [PMID: 23814495]

[10]   Askanazy M. Die Teratome nach ihrem Bau, ihrem Verlauf, ihrer Genese and im Vergleich zum experimentellen Teratoid. Verhandlungen der Deutschen Pathologischen Gesellschaft 1907; 11: 39-82.

[11] Kleinsmith LJ, Pierce GB Jr. Multipotentiality of Single Embryonal Carcinoma Cells. Cancer Res 1964; 24: 1544-51.
[PMID: 14234000]

[12] Furth JK. M. C. The transmission of leukaemia of mice with a single cell. Am J Cancer 1937; 31: 276-82.

[13] Lapidot T, Sirard C, Vormoor J, *et al.* A cell initiating human acute myeloid leukaemia after transplantation into SCID mice. Nature 1994; 367(6464): 645-8.
[http://dx.doi.org/10.1038/367645a0] [PMID: 7509044]

[14] Pierce GB, Wallace C. Differentiation of malignant to benign cells. Cancer Res 1971; 31(2): 127-34.
[PMID: 5545265]

[15] Goodman LS, Wintrobe MM, *et al.* Nitrogen mustard therapy; use of methyl-bis (beta-chloroethyl) amine hydrochloride and tris (beta-chloroethyl) amine hydrochloride for Hodgkin's disease, lymphosarcoma, leukemia and certain allied and miscellaneous disorders. J Am Med Assoc 1946; 132: 126-32.
[http://dx.doi.org/10.1001/jama.1946.02870380008004] [PMID: 20997191]

[16] Flesken-Nikitin A, Hwang CI, Cheng CY, Michurina TV, Enikolopov G, Nikitin AY. Ovarian surface epithelium at the junction area contains a cancer-prone stem cell niche. Nature 2013; 495(7440): 241-5.
[http://dx.doi.org/10.1038/nature11979] [PMID: 23467088]

[17] Chen J, Li Y, Yu TS, *et al.* A restricted cell population propagates glioblastoma growth after chemotherapy. Nature 2012; 488(7412): 522-6.
[http://dx.doi.org/10.1038/nature11287] [PMID: 22854781]

[18] Schepers AG, Snippert HJ, Stange DE, *et al.* Lineage tracing reveals Lgr5+ stem cell activity in mouse intestinal adenomas. Science 2012; 337(6095): 730-5.
[http://dx.doi.org/10.1126/science.1224676] [PMID: 22855427]

[19] Hwang RF, Moore T, Arumugam T, *et al.* Cancer-associated stromal fibroblasts promote pancreatic tumor progression. Cancer Res 2008; 68(3): 918-26.
[http://dx.doi.org/10.1158/0008-5472.CAN-07-5714] [PMID: 18245495]

[20] Xu Z, Vonlaufen A, Phillips PA, *et al.* Role of pancreatic stellate cells in pancreatic cancer metastasis. Am J Pathol 2010; 177(5): 2585-96.
[http://dx.doi.org/10.2353/ajpath.2010.090899] [PMID: 20934972]

[21] Knelson EH, Gaviglio AL, Nee JC, *et al.* Stromal heparan sulfate differentiates neuroblasts to suppress neuroblastoma growth. J Clin Invest 2014; 124(7): 3016-31.
[http://dx.doi.org/10.1172/JCI74270] [PMID: 24937430]

[22] Knelson EH, Gaviglio AL, Tewari AK, Armstrong MB, Mythreye K, Blobe GC. Type III TGF-β receptor promotes FGF2-mediated neuronal differentiation in neuroblastoma. J Clin Invest 2013; 123(11): 4786-98.
[http://dx.doi.org/10.1172/JCI69657] [PMID: 24216509]

[23] Al-Hajj M, Wicha MS, Benito-Hernandez A, Morrison SJ, Clarke MF. Prospective identification of tumorigenic breast cancer cells. Proc Natl Acad Sci USA 2003; 100(7): 3983-8.

[http://dx.doi.org/10.1073/pnas.0530291100] [PMID: 12629218]

[24]   Vaillant F, Asselin-Labat ML, Shackleton M, Forrest NC, Lindeman GJ, Visvader JE. The mammary progenitor marker CD61/beta3 integrin identifies cancer stem cells in mouse models of mammary tumorigenesis. Cancer Res 2008; 68(19): 7711-7.
[http://dx.doi.org/10.1158/0008-5472.CAN-08-1949] [PMID: 18829523]

[25]   Chen MS, Woodward WA, Behbod F, *et al.* Wnt/beta-catenin mediates radiation resistance of Sca1+ progenitors in an immortalized mammary gland cell line. J Cell Sci 2007; 120(Pt 3): 468-77.
[http://dx.doi.org/10.1242/jcs.03348] [PMID: 17227796]

[26]   Singh SK, Clarke ID, Terasaki M, *et al.* Identification of a cancer stem cell in human brain tumors. Cancer Res 2003; 63(18): 5821-8.
[PMID: 14522905]

[27]   Vaillant F, Asselin-Labat ML, Shackleton M, Forrest NC, Lindeman GJ, Visvader JE. The mammary progenitor marker CD61/beta3 integrin identifies cancer stem cells in mouse models of mammary tumorigenesis. Cancer Res 2008; 68(19): 7711-7.
[http://dx.doi.org/10.1158/0008-5472.CAN-08-1949] [PMID: 18829523]

[28]   Kozovska Z, Gabrisova V, Kucerova L. Colon cancer: Cancer stem cells markers, drug resistance and treatment. Biomedicine & Pharmacotherapy 2014; 68(8): 911-6.

[29]   Liao J, Qian F, Tchabo N, *et al.* Ovarian cancer spheroid cells with stem cell-like properties contribute to tumor generation, metastasis and chemotherapy resistance through hypoxia-resistant metabolism. PLoS One 2014; 9(1): e84941.
[http://dx.doi.org/10.1371/journal.pone.0084941] [PMID: 24409314]

[30]   Guo W, Keckesova Z, Donaher JL, *et al.* Slug and Sox9 cooperatively determine the mammary stem cell state. Cell 2012; 148(5): 1015-28.
[http://dx.doi.org/10.1016/j.cell.2012.02.008] [PMID: 22385965]

[31]   Gupta PB, Kuperwasser C, Brunet JP, *et al.* The melanocyte differentiation program predisposes to metastasis after neoplastic transformation. Nat Genet 2005; 37(10): 1047-54.
[http://dx.doi.org/10.1038/ng1634] [PMID: 16142232]

[32]   Warburg O, Wind F, Negelein E. The metabolism of tumors in the body. J Gen Physiol 1927; 8(6): 519-30.
[http://dx.doi.org/10.1085/jgp.8.6.519]

[33]   Ciavardelli D, Rossi C, Barcaroli D, *et al.* Breast cancer stem cells rely on fermentative glycolysis and are sensitive to 2-deoxyglucose treatment. Cell Death Dis 2014; 5: e1336.
[http://dx.doi.org/10.1038/cddis.2014.285] [PMID: 25032859]

[34]   Kocabas F, Zheng J, Zhang C, Sadek H. Methods in molecular biology. Hematopoietic Stem Cell Protocols. New York: Springer 2014; 1185: pp. 155-64.

[35]   Takubo K, Nagamatsu G, Kobayashi CI, *et al.* Regulation of glycolysis by Pdk functions as a metabolic checkpoint for cell cycle quiescence in hematopoietic stem cells. Cell Stem Cell 2013; 12(1): 49-61.
[http://dx.doi.org/10.1016/j.stem.2012.10.011] [PMID: 23290136]

[36]   Liu W, Beck BH, Vaidya KS, *et al.* Metastasis suppressor KISS1 seems to reverse the Warburg effect

by enhancing mitochondrial biogenesis. Cancer Res 2014; 74(3): 954-63.
[http://dx.doi.org/10.1158/0008-5472.CAN-13-1183] [PMID: 24351292]

[37] Wang Y-H, Israelsen WJ, Lee D, *et al.* Cell-state-specific metabolic dependency in hematopoiesis and leukemogenesis. Cell 2014; 158(6): 1309-23.
[http://dx.doi.org/10.1016/j.cell.2014.07.048] [PMID: 25215489]

[38] Eccles SA, Welch DR. Metastasis: recent discoveries and novel treatment strategies. Lancet 2007; 369(9574): 1742-57.
[http://dx.doi.org/10.1016/S0140-6736(07)60781-8] [PMID: 17512859]

[39] Fidler IJ. Metastasis: quantitative analysis of distribution and fate of tumor emboli labeled with 125 I-5-iodo-2'-deoxyuridine. J Natl Cancer Inst 1970; 45(4): 773-82.
[PMID: 5513503]

[40] Miele ME, Robertson G, Lee JH, *et al.* Metastasis suppressed, but tumorigenicity and local invasiveness unaffected, in the human melanoma cell line MelJuSo after introduction of human chromosomes 1 or 6. Mol Carcinog 1996; 15(4): 284-99.
[http://dx.doi.org/10.1002/(SICI)1098-2744(199604)15:4<284::AID-MC6>3.0.CO;2-G]   [PMID: 8634087]

[41] Crocetti E, Paci E. Malignant carcinoids in the USA, SEER 1992-1999. An epidemiological study with 6830 cases. Eur J Cancer Prev 2003; 12(3): 191-4.

[42] Levy AD, Sobin LH. Gastrointestinal Carcinoids: Imaging Features with Clinicopathologic Comparison 1. Radiographics 2007; 27(1): 237-57.

[43] Colombo C, Foo WC, Whiting D, *et al.* FAP-related desmoid tumors: a series of 44 patients evaluated in a cancer referral center. Histol Histopathol 2012; 27(5): 641-9.
[PMID: 22419028]

[44] Chaffer CL, Thompson EW, Williams ED. Mesenchymal to epithelial transition in development and disease. Cells Tissues Organs (Print) 2007; 185(1-3): 7-19.
[http://dx.doi.org/10.1159/000101298] [PMID: 17587803]

[45] Canesin G, Cuevas EP, Santos V, *et al.* Lysyl oxidase-like 2 (LOXL2) and E47 EMT factor: novel partners in E-cadherin repression and early metastasis colonization. Oncogene 2015; 34(8): 951-64.
[http://dx.doi.org/10.1038/onc.2014.23] [PMID: 24632622]

[46] Cheung M, Chaboissier MC, Mynett A, Hirst E. The transcriptional control of trunk neural crest induction, survival, and delamination. Developmental cell 2005; 8(2): 179-92.
[http://dx.doi.org/10.1016/j.devcel.2004.12.010]

[47] Bleul CC, Fuhlbrigge RC, Casasnovas JM, Aiuti A, Springer TA. A highly efficacious lymphocyte chemoattractant, stromal cell-derived factor 1 (SDF-1). J Exp Med 1996; 184(3): 1101-9.
[http://dx.doi.org/10.1084/jem.184.3.1101] [PMID: 9064327]

[48] Lévesque J-P, Hendy J, Takamatsu Y, Simmons PJ, Bendall LJ. Disruption of the CXCR4/CXCL12 chemotactic interaction during hematopoietic stem cell mobilization induced by GCSF or cyclophosphamide. J Clin Invest 2003; 111(2): 187-96.
[http://dx.doi.org/10.1172/JCI15994] [PMID: 12531874]

[49] Müller A, Homey B, Soto H, *et al.* Involvement of chemokine receptors in breast cancer metastasis.

Nature 2001; 410(6824): 50-6.
[http://dx.doi.org/10.1038/35065016] [PMID: 11242036]

[50]   DeCastro AJ, Cherukuri P, Balboni A, DiRenzo J. ΔNP63α Transcriptionally Activates Chemokine Receptor 4 (CXCR4) Expression to Regulate Breast Cancer Stem Cell Activity and Chemotaxis. Mol Cancer Ther 2014.
[http://dx.doi.org/10.1158/1535-7163.MCT-14-0194] [PMID: 25376609]

[51]   Mani SA, Guo W, Liao MJ, *et al.* The epithelial-mesenchymal transition generates cells with properties of stem cells. Cell 2008; 133(4): 704-15.
[http://dx.doi.org/10.1016/j.cell.2008.03.027] [PMID: 18485877]

[52]   Yang J, Mani SA, Donaher JL, *et al.* Twist, a master regulator of morphogenesis, plays an essential role in tumor metastasis. Cell 2004; 117(7): 927-39.
[http://dx.doi.org/10.1016/j.cell.2004.06.006] [PMID: 15210113]

[53]   Zhou G, Wang J, Zhao M, *et al.* Gain-of-function mutant p53 promotes cell growth and cancer cell metabolism *via* inhibition of AMPK activation. Mol Cell 2014; 54(6): 960-74.
[http://dx.doi.org/10.1016/j.molcel.2014.04.024] [PMID: 24857548]

[54]   Marie-Egyptienne DT, Lohse I, Hill RP. Cancer stem cells, the epithelial to mesenchymal transition (EMT) and radioresistance: potential role of hypoxia. Cancer Lett 2013; 341(1): 63-72.
[http://dx.doi.org/10.1016/j.canlet.2012.11.019] [PMID: 23200673]

[55]   Mujcic H, Hill RP, Koritzinsky M, Wouters BG. Hypoxia signaling and the metastatic phenotype. Curr Mol Med 2014; 14(5): 565-79.
[http://dx.doi.org/10.2174/1566524014666140603115831] [PMID: 24894165]

[56]   Tarin D, Thompson EW, Newgreen DF. The fallacy of epithelial mesenchymal transition in neoplasia. Cancer research 2008; 65(14): 5996-6001.
[http://dx.doi.org/10.1158/0008-5472.CAN-05-0699]

[57]   Ocaña OH, Córcoles R, Fabra A, *et al.* Metastatic colonization requires the repression of the epithelial-mesenchymal transition inducer Prrx1. Cancer Cell 2012; 22(6): 709-24.
[http://dx.doi.org/10.1016/j.ccr.2012.10.012] [PMID: 23201163]

[58]   Liu S, *et al.* Hedgehog signaling and Bmi-1 regulate self-renewal of normal and malignant human mammary stem cells. Cancer research 2006; 66(12): 6063-71.
[http://dx.doi.org/10.1158/0008-5472.CAN-06-0054]

[59]   Maynard MA, Ferretti R, Hilgendorf KI, Perret C, Whyte P, Lees JA. Bmi1 is required for tumorigenesis in a mouse model of intestinal cancer. Oncogene 2014; 33(28): 3742-7.
[http://dx.doi.org/10.1038/onc.2013.333] [PMID: 23955081]

[60]   Hartwell KA, Muir B, Reinhardt F, Carpenter AE, Sgroi DC, Weinberg RA. The Spemann organizer gene, Goosecoid, promotes tumor metastasis. Proc Natl Acad Sci USA 2006; 103(50): 18969-74.
[http://dx.doi.org/10.1073/pnas.0608636103] [PMID: 17142318]

[61]   Kantara C, O'Connell MR, Luthra G, *et al.* Methods for detecting circulating cancer stem cells (CCSCs) as a novel approach for diagnosis of colon cancer relapse/metastasis. Lab Invest 2015; 95(1): 100-12.
[http://dx.doi.org/10.1038/labinvest.2014.133] [PMID: 25347154]

[62] Weygant N, Qu D, May R, *et al.* DCLK1 is a broadly dysregulated target against epithelial-mesenchymal transition, focal adhesion, and stemness in clear cell renal carcinoma. Oncotarget 2015; 6(4): 2193-205.
[http://dx.doi.org/10.18632/oncotarget.3059] [PMID: 25605241]

[63] Schofield R. The relationship between the spleen colony-forming cell and the haemopoietic stem cell. Blood Cells 1978; 4(1-2): 7-25.
[PMID: 747780]

[64] Li L, Xie T. Stem cell niche: structure and function. Annu Rev Cell Dev Biol 2005; 21: 605-31.
[http://dx.doi.org/10.1146/annurev.cellbio.21.012704.131525] [PMID: 16212509]

[65] Li L, Neaves WB. Normal stem cells and cancer stem cells: the niche matters. Cancer Res 2006; 66(9): 4553-7.
[http://dx.doi.org/10.1158/0008-5472.CAN-05-3986] [PMID: 16651403]

[66] Folkins C, Man S, Xu P, Shaked Y, Hicklin DJ, Kerbel RS. s Cancer Res 2007; 67(8): 3560-4.
[http://dx.doi.org/10.1158/0008-5472.CAN-06-4238] [PMID: 17440065]

[67] Borovski T, De Sousa E Melo F, Vermeulen L, Medema JP. Cancer stem cell niche: the place to be. Cancer Res 2011; 71(3): 634-9.
[http://dx.doi.org/10.1158/0008-5472.CAN-10-3220] [PMID: 21266356]

[68] Hovinga KE, Shimizu F, Wang R, *et al.* Inhibition of notch signaling in glioblastoma targets cancer stem cells *via* an endothelial cell intermediate. Stem Cells 2010; 28(6): 1019-29.
[http://dx.doi.org/10.1002/stem.429] [PMID: 20506127]

[69] Kaplan RN, Psaila B, Lyden D. Niche-to-niche migration of bone-marrow-derived cells. Trends Mol Med 2007; 13(2): 72-81.
[http://dx.doi.org/10.1016/j.molmed.2006.12.003] [PMID: 17197241]

[70] Kaplan RN, Riba RD, Zacharoulis S, *et al.* VEGFR1-positive haematopoietic bone marrow progenitors initiate the pre-metastatic niche. Nature 2005; 438(7069): 820-7.
[http://dx.doi.org/10.1038/nature04186] [PMID: 16341007]

[71] Wang H, Yu C, Gao X, *et al.* The osteogenic niche promotes early-stage bone colonization of disseminated breast cancer cells. Cancer Cell 2015; 27(2): 193-210.
[http://dx.doi.org/10.1016/j.ccell.2014.11.017] [PMID: 25600338]

[72] Peinado H, Alečković M, Lavotshkin S, *et al.* Melanoma exosomes educate bone marrow progenitor cells toward a pro-metastatic phenotype through MET. Nat Med 2012; 18(6): 883-91.
[http://dx.doi.org/10.1038/nm.2753] [PMID: 22635005]

[73] Brown R, Curry E, Magnani L, Wilhelm-Benartzi CS, Borley J. Poised epigenetic states and acquired drug resistance in cancer. Nat Rev Cancer 2014; 14(11): 747-53.
[http://dx.doi.org/10.1038/nrc3819] [PMID: 25253389]

[74] Nowell PC. The clonal evolution of tumor cell populations. Science 1976; 194(4260): 23-8.
[http://dx.doi.org/10.1126/science.959840] [PMID: 959840]

[75] Dear TN, Kefford RF. Molecular oncogenetics of metastasis. Mol Aspects Med 1990; 11(4): 243-324.
[http://dx.doi.org/10.1016/0098-2997(90)90005-M] [PMID: 2137550]

[76]   Brableta T, Hlubek F, Spaderna S, *et al.* Invasion and metastasis in colorectal cancer: epithelial-mesenchymal transition, mesenchymal-epithelial transition, stem cells and beta-catenin. Cells Tissues Organs (Print) 2005; 179(1-2): 56-65.
       [http://dx.doi.org/10.1159/000084509] [PMID: 15942193]

[77]   Kaplan RN, Psaila B, Lyden D. Bone marrow cells in the 'pre-metastatic niche': within bone and beyond. Cancer Metastasis Rev 2006; 25(4): 521-9.
       [http://dx.doi.org/10.1007/s10555-006-9036-9] [PMID: 17186383]

CHAPTER 2

Regulation of Cell Surface Glycan Expression in Cancer Stem Cells

Reiji Kannagi[1,2,*], Bi-He Cai[1], Hsiang-Chi Huang[1] and Keiichiro Sakuma[3]

[1] *The Institute of Biomedical Sciences (IBMS), Academia Sinica, Taipei, Taiwan*

[2] *Advanced Medical Research Center, Aichi Medical University, Nagakute, Aichi, Japan*

[3] *Division of Molecular Pathology, Aichi Cancer Center, Nagoya, Aichi, Japan*

Abstract: Cell surface glycans are recognized to be good markers for human pluripotent embryonic stem cells. Typical glycan markers for human embryonic stem cells include SSEA-3, SSEA-4, TRA-1-60 and SSEA-5. Some of these glycans are recently known to be frequently expressed in human cancers, especially in cancer stem cells. Cell surface glycans undergo drastic changes also during malignant transformation, and the glycans which preferentially appear in cancers are clinically utilized as diagnostic markers for human cancers. Such tumor marker glycans include sialyl Lewis A and sialyl Lewis X, expression of which we recently showed to be enhanced in cancer stem-like cells that had undergone epithelial-mesenchymal transition. Sialyl Lewis A was also shown to be expressed in human embryonic stem cells, and to behave as an embryonic stem cell specific marker. Thus, a glycan initially described as a cancer-associated glycan in the cancer research field is now known to be an embryonic stem cell marker, while glycans formerly regarded to be typical embryonic stem cell markers in the embryology field are now shown to be cancer stem cell markers. This suggests the presence of a common induction mechanism for these glycans shared by embryonic stem cells and cancer stem cells. However, the regulatory mechanisms for stem-cell specific glycan expression remain largely unknown. In this chapter we will introduce how glycan-related genes responsible for synthesis of the stem-cell specific glycans are regulated through specific epigenetic modification, by niche-associated microenvironmental factors such as hypoxia, and during a morphogenic process like epithelial-mesenchymal transition.

***** **Corresponding author Reiji Kannagi:** The Institute of Biomedical Sciences (IBMS), Academia Sinica, 128 Sec. 2, Academia Rd. Nankang, Taipei, 11529, Taiwan, R.O.C.; Tel/Fax: +886-2-2652-3976; Email: rkannagi@ibms.sinica.edu.tw.

Keywords: Cancer stem cells, DNA methylation, Dupan-2, Embryonic stem (ES) cells, Epigenetic silencing, Epithelial-mesenchymal transition (EMT), Histone deacetylation, Histone methylation, Hypoxia inducible factor, Selectins, Sialyl Lewis A, Sialyl Lewis X, Siglecs, SLC26A2, SSEA-3, SSEA-4, SSEA-5, ST6GalNAc6, Sulfate transporter, TRA-1-60.

INTRODUCTION

Perhaps the most important premise assumed in the theory of cancer stem cells is that they are derived from normal stem cells in the given tissue where the process of carcinogenesis takes place. If this is true, the cancer cells may inherit remnants of epigenetic patterns of gene expression from the normal stem cells through the epigenetic memory, and may share with them the common microenvironments which are termed as niche *in toto*, and will actively undergo extensive morphologic changes such as EMT/MET required for "organogenesis," which may be represented as "metastasis" in the case of cancer cells. Of course the behavior of cancer stem cells will not be exactly the same as normal stem cells, as the cancer stem cells will exhibit novel features that will be acquired through the reprogramming process during the course of carcinogenesis. It is conceivable that although cancer initiating cells originate from normal tissue stem cells in the given organs, there is still not solid evidence indicating that the origin of cancer initiating cells is strictly confined to normal stem cells in every tissue and organ. Therefore, the terms "tumor-initiating cell," "tumor-propagating cells" or "cancer stem-like cell" are sometimes recommended instead of cancer stem cell. There is, however, no doubt that the concept of cancer stem cells has significantly contributed to our understanding of many biological aspects of cancers.

CANCER STEM CELLS AND EPIGENETIC SILENCING OF GLYCOGENES

Induction of Typical Cancer-associated Glycans Through Epigenetic Silencing of Glycan-related Genes Responsible for Synthesis of Normal Glycans

It has long been known that glycans undergo drastic changes upon carcinogenesis. The glycans preferentially appear in cancer cells, such as sialyl Lewis A and sialyl

Lewis X, are utilized in clinical diagnosis of cancers. We recently showed that expression of these cancer-associated glycans is induced in cancer cells at the early stages of carcinogenesis through epigenetic silencing of several glycan-related genes responsible for synthesis of normal glycans.

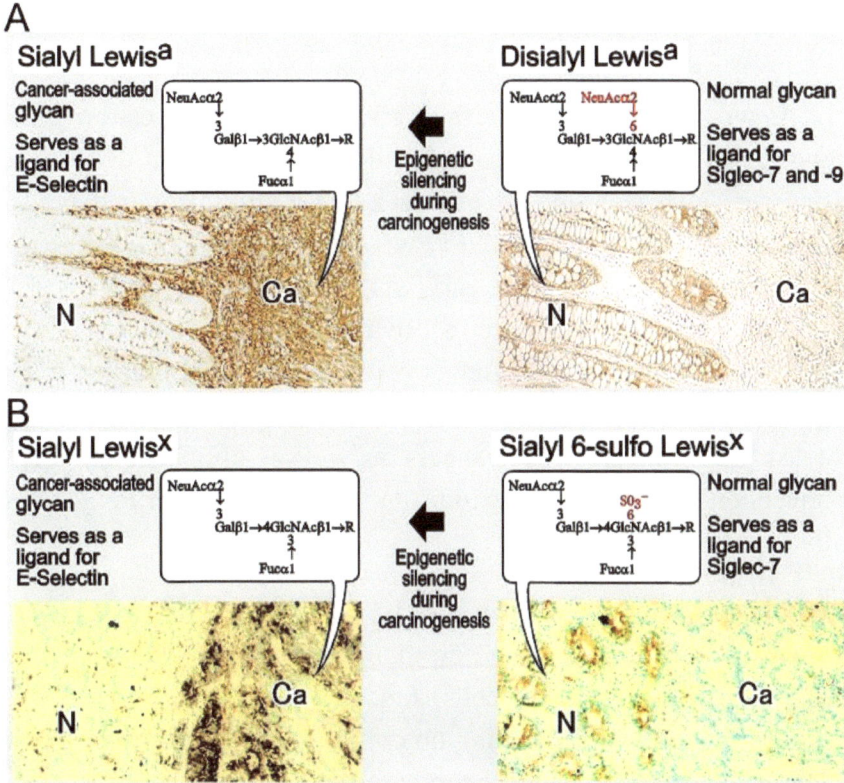

Fig. (1). Examples of interconversion of normal glycans into cancer-associated glycans. Panel **A**, transition of normal glycan, disialyl Lewis A, to cancer-associated glycan, sialyl Lewis A, upon malignant transformation. Panel **B**, conversion of normal glycan, sialyl 6-sulfo Lewis X to a cancer-associated glycan, sialyl Lewis X glycan upon malignant transformation. Typical distribution patterns shown were obtained by immunohistochemical staining using specific anti-glycan antibodies of consecutive sections prepared from colon cancer tissues. Ca, cancer cells; N, non-malignant epithelial cells. (Adapted from references [5 - 7]).

A variety of glycans are expressed in normal epithelial cells, expression of some of which is conventional in that they are also constitutively expressed in cancers. In contrast, some other normal glycans exhibit preferential expression in non-malignant epithelial cells, and tend to decrease or disappear and be replaced by cancer-associated glycans upon malignant transformation. Such normal glycans include disialyl Lewis A, which was found to be preferentially expressed in non-malignant epithelial cells of the digestive organs (Fig. **1A**) [1 - 4], and its clinical evaluation in patients' sera was proposed to be clinically useful for differential diagnoses of benign and malignant diseases, especially when routine serum determination of sialyl Lewis A, a widely applied serum marker for cancers, gave false-positive results [1 - 4].

The disialyl Lewis A glycan is a normal counterpart of the cancer-associated glycan, sialyl Lewis A, and soon epigenetic silencing of *ST6GalNAc6*, a gene for α2,6sialyltransferase, was found to be the key for diminishing expression of disialyl Lewis A and induction of sialyl Lewis A in cancers [5]. Down-regulation of *ST6GalNAc6* was observed at the early stages of colon carcinogenesis in the normal-adenoma-carcinoma sequence [8]. In addition to the cancers of digestive organs, preferential loss of disialyl Lewis A expression is also noted in prostate cancers [9], and cancer-associated decrease of the *ST6GalNAc6* mRNA level is noted in breast [10] and renal [11] cancers, as well as glioblastoma [12]. Thus, this interconversion of glycans seems to be applicable to a wider range of cancers than initially expected.

Another example of a "normal" glycan is sialyl 6-sulfo Lewis X, which was found to be also preferentially expressed in non-malignant epithelial cells of the colon, and to disappear in colonic cancer cells (Fig. **1B**) [5]. This finding was in line with the classical histochemical finding on colon cancer glycans that the amount of sulfomucin is decreased in cancers compared to non-malignant colonic tissues [13]. Sialyl 6-sulfo Lewis X glycan is a normal counterpart of the well-known cancer-associated glycan, sialyl Lewis X. Epigenetic silencing of *SLC26A2*, a gene for sulfate transporter DTDST, was found to be a key mechanism responsible for diminished expression of sialyl 6-sulfo Lewis X and appearance of sialyl Lewis X in cancers [14]. Down-regulation of *SLC26A2* was observed at the early stages of colon carcinogenesis. The results of DNA microarray analyses on the microdissected cells from polyps with malignant transformation indicated that transcription of *SLC26A2* is already decreased in colonic polyps, and exhibits continuous down-regulation along with the entire normal-adenoma-carcinoma sequence [15]. It is notable that not only the genes for glycosyltransferases, which are directly involved in glycan synthesis, but also those for some transporters or enzymes in the intermediate carbohydrate metabolism, are capable of playing a key role in the cancer-associated glycan alteration.

The normal glycans, disialyl Lewis A and sialyl 6-sulfo Lewis X, serve as ligands for Siglec-7 or -9, which are immunosuppressive glycan-recognition molecules having immunosuppressive ITIM motifs in their cytoplasmic domains, and are expressed by a variety of immune cells including tissue macrophages in the normal mucosal membrane [6, 16]. Ligation of either Siglec-7 or Siglec-9 had suppressive effects on production of COX2 and IL-12 by macrophage-like cells [16]. COX2 is a pro-inflammatory molecule known to promote cancer progression [17], and therefore Siglec-7 and Siglec-9 behave as anti-oncogenic molecules. Based on these results, it was proposed that normal glycans may play a role in maintaining immunological homeostasis and preventing cancer progression. The loss of these normal glycans due to epigenetic silencing of the key genes, *ST6GalNAc6* and *SLC26A2*, upon malignant transformation is expected to further facilitate carcinogenesis.

Another biological function of the normal glycans is their association with cell proliferation status. For instance, the decreased transcription of *SLC26A2* in cancers mediates the loss of normal glycan sialyl 6-sulfo Lewis X and induction of cancer-associated glycan sialyl Lewis X, and at the same time strongly induces cell proliferation [14]. The suppressive effect of the *SLC26A2* gene on cell proliferation was clearly reproduced in experiments using a Tet-off expression vector for *SLC26A2* [14]. It is not clear whether or not the growth suppression conferred by this gene is due to its effects on glycan sulfation, because *SLC26A2* is a sulfate transporter gene which can affect not only glycan sulfation but also sulfation of other molecules such as proteins and lipids. Still, it can at least be proposed that this is an example indicating the close link between change in glycan expression and cell proliferation status.

Mechanisms for Epigenetic Silencing of Glycan-related Genes During the Course of Carcinogenesis

Aberrant DNA methylation at promoter CpG islands is one of the most common and well-established epigenetic abnormalities in cancer. A classical example of this is DNA methylation of A- and B-enzymes in cancers, which was shown to explain cancer-associated decrease of normal A- and B-blood type glycan expressions in a variety of human cancers [18, 19]. Loss of the Sd^a blood group substance in colon cancers was also shown to be due to DNA methylation of the *B4GALNT2* gene promotor [20]. The decrease in all these glycan epitopes attached to the lactosamine or polylactosamine backbone structures is proposed to indirectly facilitate expression of cancer-associated glycan epitopes such as sialyl Lewis A and sialyl Lewis X, synthesized from common precursors, by leaving the surplus substrates for the enzymes responsible for synthesis of the latter two cancer-associated glycans [21, 22].

There are many examples of genes involved in glycan synthesis which are regulated by DNA methylation in cancers. *HS3ST2* (*3OST2*) is a typical example of genes long known to be strongly hypermethylated in a variety of cancers [23], and is sometimes utilized even as a positive control in DNA methylation analyses. The biological significance of this gene was not known until the heparan sulfate 3-*O*-sulfotransferase encoded by this gene was recently reported to suppress cell proliferation and migration [24]. The exact mechanisms behind these observed phenomena await further investigation, but this is an indication of another link between cancer cell proliferation and glycan expression, especially their sulfate modification. The roles of heparan sulfates as extracellular co-receptors for growth factors have been well documented [25].

Histone modification is also intimately involved in cancer-associated epigenetic silencing of glycan-related genes. Transcription of *ST6GalNAc6* was initially reported to be recovered either by treatment with histone deacetylation inhibitor or DNA methylation inhibitor [6], but the results of subsequent experiments indicated histone modification to be the most frequent mechanism for silencing of this gene. Histone modification was also proposed to be the major mechanism for epigenetic silencing of the sulfate transporter gene *SLC26A2*, and in the case of this gene, significant participation of histone trimethylation at H3K27 was suspected in addition to histone deacetylation [14] (Fig. **2**). Accordingly, addition of not only HDAC inhibitors, but histone methyltransferase inhibitor DZNep, was shown to stoichiometrically induce *SLC26A2* transcription (Fig. **2**). Participation of DNA methylation in cancer- associated suppression of this gene was recently reported for papillary thyroid cancers [26]. Our recent results indicated that DZNep induce also ST6GalNAc6, indicating histone trimethylation at H3K27 by the methyltransferase EZH2 figures heavily in epigenetic silencing of normal glycan-related genes and induction of cancer-associated glycans. Regulation of gene expression through H3K27me3 is shown to play a pivotal role in carcinogenesis of the colon [27, 28] as well as other tissues and organs, and association of EZH2 with malignant characteristics is noted.

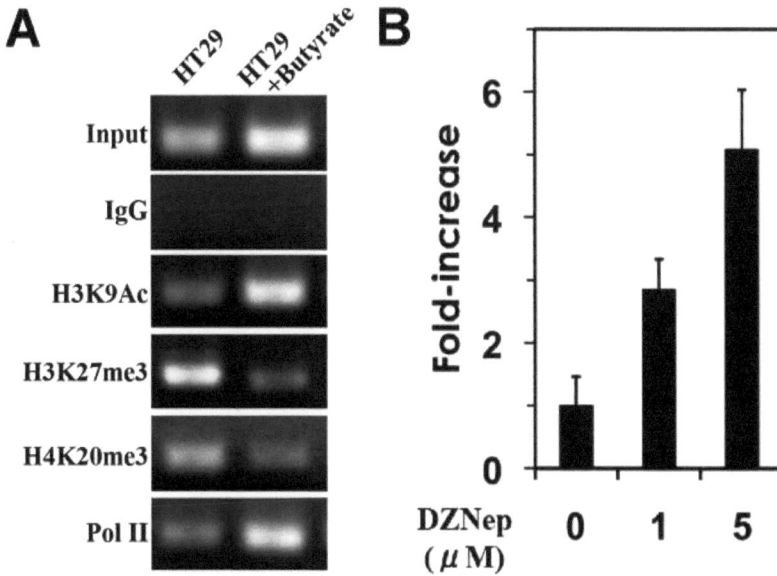

Fig. (2). Epigenetic silencing of *SLC26A2* gene in colon cancer cells. Panel **A**, results of ChIP assays in human colon cancer HT29 cells cultured with or without an HDAC inhibitor, butyrate. Panel **B**, effect of histone methyltransferase inhibitor DZNep on the transcription level of the *SLC26A2* gene. (Adapted from reference [14]).

Almost three decades ago, we had classified the cancer-associated changes of glycan expression into two categories; one had been "incomplete synthesis" of normal glycans, and the other "*neo*synthesis" of abnormal glycans [29]. The concept of "incomplete synthesis" had referred to the accumulation of structurally simpler abnormal glycans due to disturbance of synthetic pathways for normal glycans, which mainly occurs during the course of early carcinogenesis. This concept assumed some suppression to occur in the transcription/translation of genes involved in the synthesis of normal glycans during carcinogenesis. At present, the major suppression mechanism is regarded to be epigenetic silencing [21, 22, 30]. Among the several mechanisms for epigenetic silencing, histone trimethylation at H3K27 by the methyltransferase EZH2 seems to play major roles in the induction of well-known cancer-associated glycans such as sialyl Lewis A and sialyl Lewis X. The process of "incomplete synthesis" is known to start working at relatively early stages of carcinogenesis.

Differentiation-dependent Expression of Glycans in Normal Tissue Stem Cells

Significant alteration of glycan expression is also observed when the stem cells in various tissues and organs differentiate into fully mature epithelial- or parenchymal cells. For instance, sialyl 6-sulfo Lewis X is expressed in most of the mature epithelial cells in the colon, except in the cells at the crypt base, where the cognate intestinal stem cells are known to be localized (Fig. **3A**). In contrast, sialyl Lewis X, the cancer-associated glycan, is localized in the cells at the crypt base, and is not expressed in mature colonic epithelial cells (Fig. **3B**). Although much weaker than in cancer cells, preferential expression of sialyl Lewis X in the normal crypt cells suggests that the conversion process of this glycan into the normal sialyl 6-sulfo Lewis X glycan is also suppressed in the intestinal stem cells. It is not clear at present whether the preferential expression of sialyl Lewis X in stem-like cells in the colonic crypt is due to any epigenetic silencing of the gene for sulfate transporter, *SLC26A2*, as is the case in the colon cancer cells. In this context, it is noteworthy that the DTDST protein, the product of the *SLC26A2* gene, is also expressed preferentially in mature epithelial cells in the colonic villi, but not in the cells at the crypt base (Fig. **3C**). The decrease in the expression of *SLC26A2* can be suggested to at least partially contribute to the crypt-specific expression of sialyl Lewis X in colonic epithelium. Cell surface glycans are useful markers in dissecting intestinal stem cells. Of note is that the important evidence for clonality of crypt cells derived from monoclonal intestinal stem cells came from the study of *O*-glycans carrying *O*-acetylated sialic acid as a tracing marker [31, 32].

Normal tissue stem cells can be good candidates for the origin of cancer cells, because they are generally supposed to have a long life span, thus posing a higher risk for accumulating tumorigenic mutations and self-renewing proliferative activity which enables generation of tumors. Compared to this, the normal colonic epithelial cells are known to have a lifetime of about five days, and are continuously renewed by the stem cells in the crypt; thus they do not have sufficient lifespan to accumulate enough genetic and epigenetic anomalies for malignant transformation. There is a good chance that cancer stem cells would possess stem-cell traits inherited from normal stem cells in the given tissues. The similar epigenetic mechanisms may work both in normal intestinal stem cells and in the colon cancer stem cells.

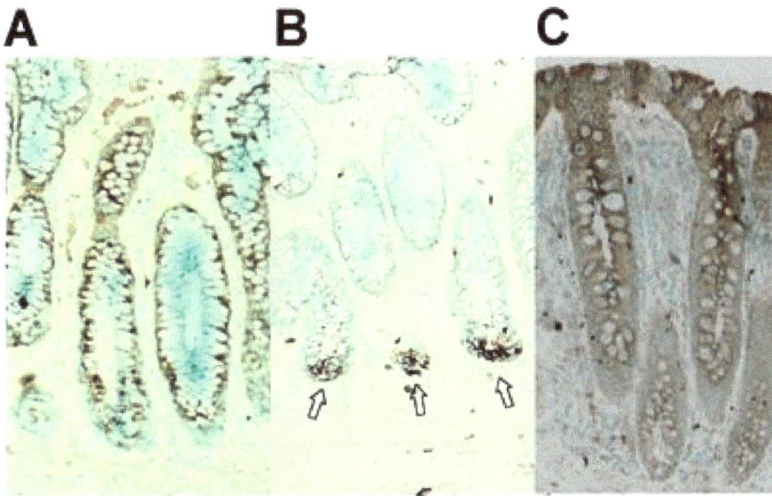

Fig. (3). Expression of normal- and cancer-associated glycans in human intestinal stem-cell like cells at the colonic crypt base. Panel **A**, expression of sialyl 6-sulfo Lewis X, and panel **B**, that of sialyl Lewis X. Note that the normal glycan, sialyl 6-sulfo Lewis X, is expressed in fully-differentiated epithelial cells, whereas expression of the cancer-associated glycan, sialyl Lewis X, is confined to crypt cells as indicated by the arrows. Panel **C**, distribution of the sulfate transporter DTDST protein encoded by the *SLC26A2* gene in differentiated epithelial cells but not in crypt cells, which is compatible with the proposition that this gene is closely involved in the differential expression of these glycans.

Histone trimethylation at H3K27 is known to play a pivotal role in differentiation of embryonic stem cells. Disruption of many genes, which encode epigenetic modifiers including EZH2, have resulted in embryonic lethality, indicating that epigenetic modifiers are important players in embryonic development [33]. Pluripotent embryonic stem cells are known to have a unique epigenetic signature compared to that of differentiated cells. Embryonic stem cells have both active histone markers such as H3K4me3 and repressive marker H3K27me3 in the regulatory regions of developmental genes, and most bivalent genes lose one of these markers and become monovalent upon differentiation [34, 35]. Bivalent chromatin marks are regulated by the functionally opposing polycomb complexes such as PRC1 and PRC2, which produce H3K27me3 modification, and MLL complexes which induce H3K4 methylation and gene transcription. EZH2 is a subunit of PRC2 having methyltransferase activity, and catalyzes H3K27 trimethylation. Intestinal stem cells may also have bivalent chromatin marks in some subsets of genes, and the genes to be expressed in differentiated cells, such as *SLC26A2* or *ST6GalNAc6*, acquire the active marker and lose the repressive marker. It is tempting to speculate that cancer stem cells inherit such epigenetic regulatory machinery from tissue stem cells and reactivate them.

Epigenetic drugs are so far not yet actively utilized for therapy of cancers, but several reports suggest them to be beneficial for chemoprevention of cancers [36, 37]. Assessment of normal glycan expression in parallel with the expression of cancer-associated glycans may be useful for monitoring therapeutic effects in such regimens. A quite obvious problem in the application of epigenetic drugs for cancer therapy is that they are directed only to epigenetic changes, and shall not correct physical genetic anomalies, such as the mutation, deletion, amplification and translocation, frequently encountered in cancers. Epigenetic silencing of a part of genes is expected to occur when the embryonic stem cells develop into more tissue-specific stem cells, and further silencing will take place when such tissue-specific stem cells differentiate into mature parenchymal cells in each organ. The embryonic stem cells are to undergo several steps of developmental epigenetic silencing. Cancer-associated silencing of a subset of genes will occur upon carcinogenesis. Another problem for epigenetic drugs is that most of them do not seem to discriminate the epigenetic silencing associated with normal development and cancer-associated epigenetic silencing, and work rather non-specifically. Developmental epigenetic silencing and cancer-associated epigenetic silencing may share many similarities. Many drugs aimed at correcting abnormal epigenetic silencing in cancers may work also on normal developmental epigenetic silencing. Activity of EZH2 or PRC2 is known to be affected by various factors, which include post-translational modification such as *O-*

GlcNAcylation [38]. An interesting remaining issue in the field would be to explore whether there are any cancer-specific factors affecting epigenetic silencing.

ENHANCED STEMNESS AND ALTERED GLYCAN EXPRESSION BY TUMOR HYPOXIA

Acquisition of Resistance to Hypoxia by Cancer Cells in Advanced Stage of Cancers

Cancer cells must cope with hypoxic environments to survive at the locally advanced stages, and some cancer cell clones having hypoxia-resistant characteristics appear through accumulation of genetic anomalies. Such hypoxia-resistant cancer cells usually exhibit a higher proliferation rate, enhanced cell mobility, greater angiogenic activity and stronger multi-drug resistance, thus having multiple advantages over other cancer cell clones, and eventually occupying all cancer cell nests. The transcription factors called hypoxia-inducible factors (HIFs), perhaps both HIF-1α and HIF-2α, play central roles when cancer cells acquire hypoxia-resistant characteristics.

Intense changes of glycan expression are observed in advanced-stage cancers partly because HIFs induce transcription of a variety of genes involved in synthesis of glycans [30, 39]. For instance, tumor hypoxia induces, through the action of HIFs, transcription of genes for sialyltransferase, fucosyltransferase and UDP-galactose transporter, which are involved in the synthesis of sialyl Lewis A and sialyl Lewis X [40]. Tumor hypoxia thus enhances expression of sialyl Lewis A and sialyl Lewis X in cancer cells, which further helps these cells cope with hypoxic environments, since these glycans serve as ligands for vascular E-selectin and mediate adhesion of cancer cells to endothelial cells. Interaction between E-selectins on endothelial cells and its ligands on cancer cells is known to facilitate tumor vascularization [41] as well as hematogenous metastasis [39]. HIFs also induce transcription of genes for several enzymes in the synthetic pathway of the lipid moiety of glycolipids, which is expected to affect their localization in cell membrane microdomains [42, 43].

The gene for a sialic acid transporter sialin, *SLC17A5*, is also induced by HIFs

[44]. Normal cells synthesize sialic acid, usually from the *de novo* synthetic pathway starting from UDP-GlcNAc. Cancer cells in general have an increased demand for sialic acids. Cancer cells seem to enhance the *de novo* synthetic pathway to some extent to meet the increased demands for sialoconjugate synthesis [45], but upon progression, cancer cells tend to rely more on the salvage pathway, which reutilizes the sialic acid residues cleaved from exogenous glycoconjugates in lysosomes. Sialin is a lysosomal sialic acid transporter that pumps in free sialic acids released in lysosomes to cytoplasm, and is closely involved in the salvage pathway. In humans, the sialic acid species provided by the *de novo* synthetic pathway is limited only to NeuAc but not NeuGc, because humans lack the enzyme which converts CMP-NeuAc, to CMP-NeuGc. On the other hand, sialic acids transported by sialin contain NeuGc, the non-human sialic acid derived from fetal calf serum under cell culture conditions and from a dietary origin under *in vivo* conditions. Consequently, the amount of glycans containing NeuGc in cancer cells having enhanced sialin activity is usually higher than that in non-malignant cells. A glycan containing NeuGc was sometimes known to be antigenic to humans, and was termed Hanganatziu-Deicher antigen. This antigen was for a long time counted as a member of cancer-associated glycans, as cancers have a higher amount of NeuGc-containing glycans than normal tissues. The Hanganatziu-Deicher antigen occurs late during cancer progression, mainly in the advanced stages of cancers, because its appearance is driven by HIF-1α, which starts to work in the advanced stages. Recently, cultured ovarian cancer cells having an extremely high NeuGc content were reported, and other mechanisms, in addition to enhanced sialin transcription, were suggested to be involved in this extremely high NeuGc expression [46].

Normal Stem Cells and Their Hypoxic Niches

It has become increasingly clear that hypoxia plays a major role in maintaining stemness of normal stem cells including embryonic stem cells. Hypoxic conditions are known to be required to maintain the full pluripotency of human embryonic stem cells. When maintained under hypoxic conditions, human ES cells exhibited increased expression of the pluripotency marker glycan SSEA-3, and transcription of c-MYC was induced [47]. Enhanced spontaneous differentiation of human ES cells is often observed at higher oxygen levels, as ascertained by a loss of OCT4 and SSEA-4 expression [48].

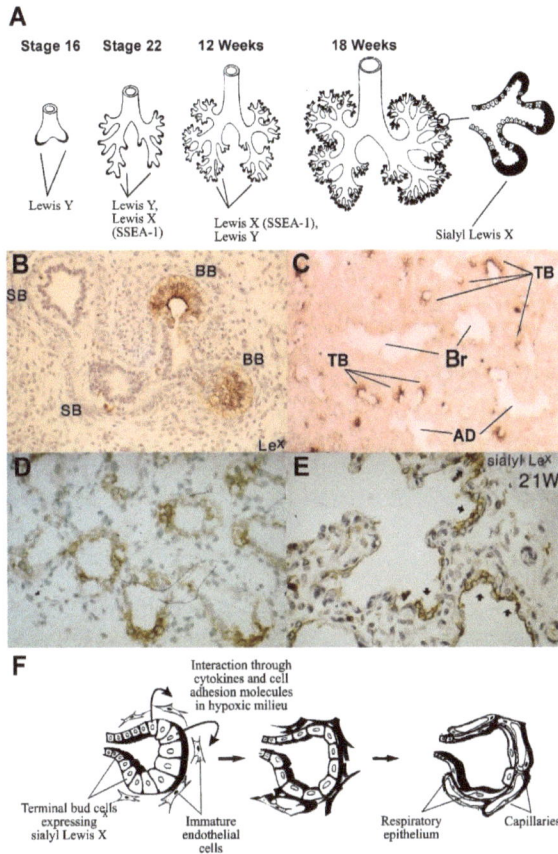

Fig. (4). Development-dependent expression of sialyl Lewis X and related glycans during human lung morphogenesis. Panel **A**, a scheme showing sequential induction of Lewis Y, Lewis X (SSEA-1), and sialyl Lewis X glycans in stem cells for each developmental stage of human lung organogenesis. Lewis Y appears in tracheal bud cells at stage 16, Lewis X in bronchial and bronchiolar bud cells, and sialyl Lewis X finally appears in terminal bud cells. Panel **B**, expression of Lewis X in bronchiolar bud cells exhibiting bifurcate branching. BB, bronchiolar bud cells; SB, stem bronchiolus. Panel **C**, expression of sialyl Lewis X in terminal bud cells. Note that it is specifically expressed in terminal bud cells (TB), but is not detected in epithelial cells of alveolar ducts (AD) and bronchioles (Br). Panel **D** shows a higher magnification of terminal bud cells expressing sialyl Lewis X at the similar stage as in panel **C**. Panel **E**, expression of sialyl Lewis X in terminal bud cells at a later stage in a 22-week-old embryo. The terminal bud cells show flattened morphology indicating progression of the maturation process, but still express sialyl Lewis X. Panel **F**, a scheme showing interaction of terminal bud cells and immature endothelial cells in the alveolus formation. Adopted from references [67, 68].

Hypoxia-inducible factors are involved in the regulation of stemness in the normal

ES cells [49], and especially HIF-2α is known to directly induce OCT4 [50], c-Myc [51], Nanog and Sox2 [52]. Oct 3/4, Sox2, Klf4, and c-Myc are regarded to be typical stem-cell associated genes, because iPS cells can be induced by the transduction of these four transcription factors [53, 54]. It was shown that hypoxia enhanced expression of transcription levels of endogenous OCT4 and Nanog, and increased the number of iPS cells bearing SSEA-3/-4 glycans during the course of iPS generation [55].

Not only embryonic stem cells, but also more specialized lineage-committed stem cells in a variety of tissues and organs also favor hypoxic conditions. It is well known that hematopoietic stem cells are specifically localized in hypoxic bone marrow microenvironments/niches [56, 57]. Hypoxia is also known to increase stemness of cardiac stem cells [58], is required for maintenance of neural progenitors [59], and for mesenchymal stem cells prepared either from bone marrow or adipose tissue [60, 61].

In some tissues, changes in oxygen concentration *per se* directly regulate differentiation and organogenesis by stem cells, such as in development of placenta, lung and cardiovascular system [49]. For instance, lung organogenesis is known to be typically guided by oxygen gradients [62 - 66]. This accompanies exquisitely elegant changes of glycan stem cell markers, such as SSEA-1 (Lewis X) and its sialylated form (sialyl Lewis X), which sequentially appear and orderly disappear along with the branching of bud cells for trachea, bronchi and bronchioles [67, 68] (Fig. **4**). Hypoxia-inducible factors are known to regulate branching morphogenesis of not only tracheal and bronchial trees [63, 69], but also that of renal tubules in the kidney [70].

In the development of the human lung, SSEA-1 glycan (Lewis X) and its fucosylated form (Lewis Y) are expressed sequentially in the tracheal, bronchial and bronchiolar bud cells, which are the stem cells for bronchial tree formation, whereas sialyl Lewis X specifically appears in the terminal bud cells, which are the stem cells at the stage of alveolar formation (Fig. **4**). These terminal bud cells grow into surrounding connective tissues forming bifurcate branching structures, and interact with endothelial cells to form respiratory alveoli. Secretion of vasculotrophic cytokines from the bud cells such as VEGF through transcriptional induction by hypoxia-inducible factor HIF-2α is known to be crucial for the process of alveolus formation [69], suggesting the importance of hypoxic environments for the morphogenesis by the stem cells. In this context, it is noteworthy that sialyl Lewis X has cell adhesion activity, and is known to mediate adhesion of epithelial cells to endothelial cells.

STEM CELLS AND GLYCAN ALTERATION IN EPITHELIO-MESENCHYMAL TRANSITION

Glycan Alteration in Epithelio-mesenchymal Transition of Cancer Cells

Cancer stem cells were initially characterized by the cell-surface markers such as CD133, CD44 and CD166 [71, 72], but their expression is dependent on the cell lines employed in the experiments. Some of the researchers seem to have preferred to analyze cancer stem cells in the context of more biological phenomena such as epithelial-mesenchymal transition (EMT). EMT is a biological process known to be governed by several well-defined transcription factors such as SNAIL, TWIST and ZEB, and the cells which have undergone EMT are known to exhibit a high similarity to those of cancer stem cells [73]. EMT is a critical event in the advanced stages of cancers which prepares cancer cells for metastasis.

Table 1. Examples of glycans and glycan-related genes reported to exhibit altered expression levels in cancer stem cells or EMT-induced cancer stem-like cells.

Glycans involved	Genes affected	Experimental design	Reference
SSEA-1 (Lewis X, CD15)	(Not described)	Tumor spheres	[97, 98]
Gg4, GM2	*B3GalT4* (decrease)	EMT induced by glycolipid synthase inhibitor, TGFβ, and hypoxia	[74, 75]
Hyaluronan	*HAS2* (increase)	EMT induced by TGFβ	[109]
Hyaluronan	*HAS2, HAS3* (increase)	EMT induced by EGF and IL-1β	[110]
I-branching in polylactosamines	*GCNT2* (increase)	EMT induced by TGFβ	[111]
Sialyl Lewis A/ Sialyl Lewis X	*ST3GAL1/3/4, FUT3* (increase); *FUT2* (decrease)	EMT induced by EGF/bFGF	[76]

(Table 1) contd.....

Glycans involved	Genes affected	Experimental design	Reference
N-glycan	*MGAT3* (decrease)	EMT induced by TGFβ	[76]
N-glycan	*MGAT3* (decrease)	EMT induced by TGFβ	[112]
O-glycan	*GCNT1* (increase)	Breast cancer tumor initiating cells	[114]
GD2	*ST8SIA1* (increase)	Cancer stem cells induced through EMT	[115]
glycolipids, Gb3	*UGCG* (increase)	Breast cancer stem cells	[116]
Hyaluronan	*HAS2* (increase)	Breast cancer stem cells	[117]
Lectin binding	*Mgat5*, *FUT8* and *β3GalT5* (increase); *Mgat3* (decrease)	EMT induced by HGF	[118]
N-glycan	*ST6GAL1* (increase)	Colon cancer stem cells	[119]
N-glycan	*FUT8* (increase)	EMT induced by TGFβ	[120]
GM3	*ST3GAL5* (increase)	EMT induced by TGFβ	[121]
GD2, GD3, GM2, GD1a	*ST3GAL5*, *B4GALNT1*, *ST8SIA1*, *ST3GAL2* (increase)	Cancer stem cells induced through EMT	[122]
N-glycans	*FUCA1*, *MAN2A1*, *NEU1*, *HEXB*, *ST6GAL1* (decrease)	EMT induced by TGFβ	[123]
α-Dystroglycan glycosylation	*LARGE2 (GYLTY1B)*, (decrease)	EMT induced by ZEB1	[124]
β1,6-GlcNAc branched N-glycans	*MGAT5* (decrease)	EMT induced by TGFβ	[125]
N-glycans	*ALG9*, *MAN2A1*, *MGAT3*, *NEU1*, *NEU2*, *MANBA* (decrease) MGAT4B (increase)	EMT induced by TGFβ	[126]
Sialoconjugates	*NEU4* (increase)	Sphere formation	[127]
Increased α1,2-/ α1,3-/ α1,4- fucosylation	*FUT1, FUT2, FUT3, FUT4, FX, GDP-Fuc Transporter* (increase)	Drug resistance and sphere formation	[128]
Sialyl Lewis X	*FUT3, FUT6* (increase)	Sphere formation	[129]
GM3	*B3GLCT*, *ST3GAL5*, *ST6GALNAC5* (decrease)	MET induced by *miR-200*	[130]

EMT was found to accompany significant alteration in the cell surface glycan expression [74 - 76, 109 - 113, 115, 118, 120 - 126]. The initial reports indicated that a decrease in the expression of glycolipids Gg4 and GM2 accompanies TGFβ-induced EMT, and this has functional relevance because the addition of an inhibitor of glycolipid synthesis induced EMT, while the addition of Gg4 and GM2 abrogated EMT [74, 75]. Since then, many instances have been reported indicating a close relationship between EMT and cell surface glycan expression. Examples of glycans and glycan-related genes which have been reported to exhibit altered transcription levels in EMT-induced cancer cells and/or cancer stem cells are listed in Table **1**.

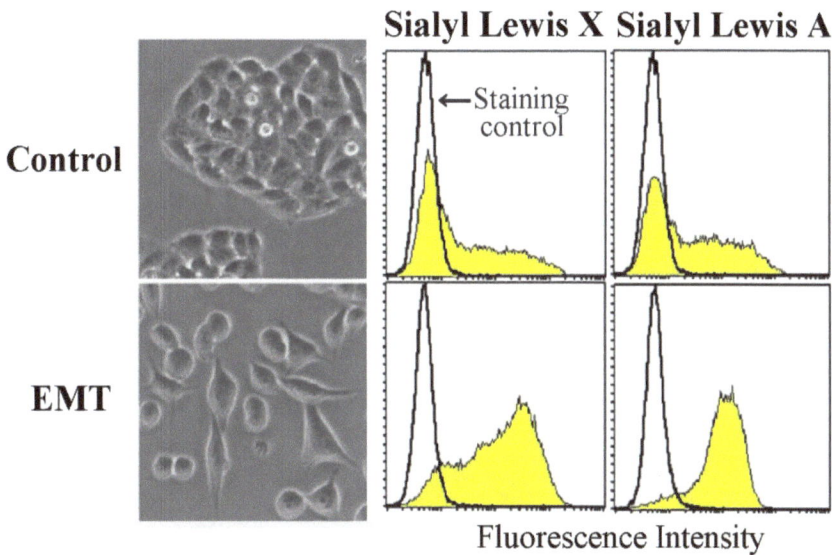

Fig. (5). Induction of cancer-associated glycans sialyl Lewis A and sialyl Lewis X in cancer cells which had undergone epithelio-mesenchymal transition (EMT). Human colon cancer cells DLD-1 were cultured with EGF/bFGF in serum-free medium to induce EMT. Morphological changes (left panel) and results of flow-cytometric analyses of sialyl Lewis A and sialyl Lewis X expression (right panel) upon EMT are shown. Adopted from reference [76].

We observed that EMT induces transcription of several genes involved in glycan synthesis, such as sialyltransferases, fucosyltransferases and galactosyltransferases, which was mediated by transcription factors c-Myc and CDX2 [75]. Consequently, cancer cells which had undergone EMT have a higher expression of well-known cancer-associated glycans, sialyl Lewis A and sialyl Lewis X (Fig. **5**), and strongly bind to vascular E-selectin. Cancer cells converted from epithelial to fibroblastic morphology with reduced E-cadherin level and enhanced sialyl Lewis glycan expression were also observed in the invasion front of the cancer tissues prepared from patient samples (Fig. **6**). Several decades ago, it had been noticed that cancer cells in the invasion front having a mesenchymal cell-like morphology frequently express these glycans strongly [77]. Judging from the recent findings mentioned above, this must have been due to the EMT-induced transcription of glycan-related genes. This also has functional relevance since sialyl Lewis A and sialyl Lewis X glycans serve as ligands for vascular E-selectin, and mediate tumor vasculogenesis and hematogenous metastasis of cancer cells [39, 41, 78 - 80]. In our experimental system, expression of sialyl Lewis A and sialyl Lewis X was enhanced in cancer cells after EMT, while a paradoxical decrease was noted in the expression of some other glycans that had also been assumed to be cancer-associated, such as Lewis Y glycan [76]. This unexpected finding suggested that some hitherto-known cancer-associated glycans, exemplified by sialyl Lewis A/X, are linked to a more malignant population of cancer cells such as cancer stem cells, while others may not be.

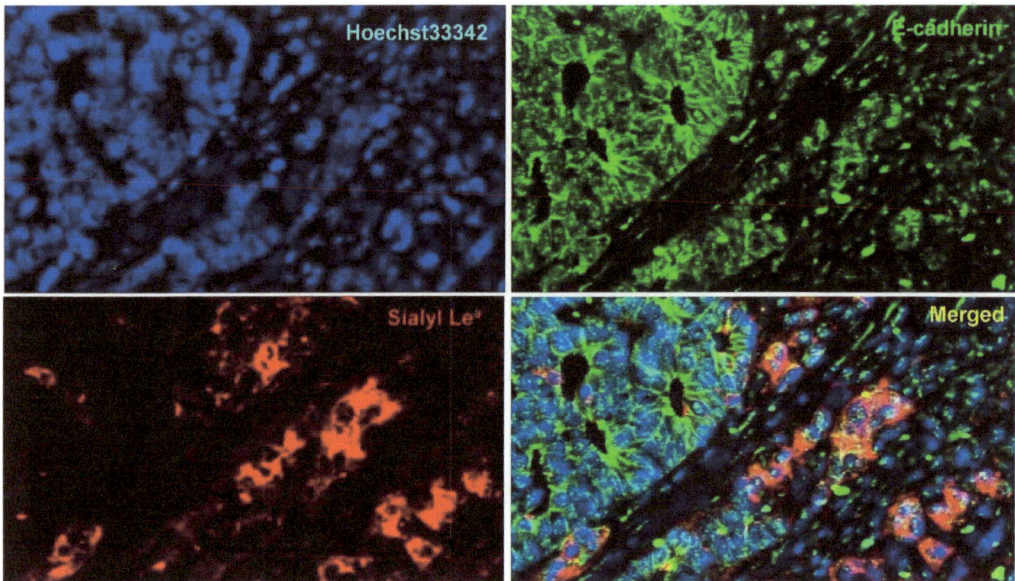

Fig. (6). Sialyl Lewis A expression on colon cancer cells undergoing EMT *in vivo*. Expression of E-cadherin (green) and sialyl Lewis A (red) was examined on a human colon cancer section by immunohistochemistry. Note that cancer cells in the infiltration front show decreased E-cadherin expression and increased sialyl Lewis A expression. Blue, staining with Hoechst 33342. Adopted from reference [76].

Normal Stem Cells and Plasticity to Undergo EMT/MET

Normal stem cells undergo multiple rounds of EMT and its reverse process, MET, during embryonic development. EMT is known to be involved in multiple steps during normal embryogenesis, including implantation, gastrulation and neural crest cell emigration [81]. The occurrence of EMT in cancers is often considered as the reactivation of similar developmental programs. However, several differences between EMT in normal development and cancers have been noted. One is that the EMT process displayed by the normal stem cells is pre-programmed and "self-contained" [82], while that in cancers is induced or deeply affected by inflammatory cells present in the cancer microenvironment by way of receiving potent EMT-promoting signals from these cells. Another difference is that EMT and MET seem to be equally important in the embryonic development, while the role of EMT is emphasized as an important mechanism to confine metastatic ability, and the role of MET is not fully clear in cancers. Cancer cells may frequently undergo EMT and show mesenchymal characteristics during the course of metastasis, but after the completion of migration, every surgical pathologist knows that the cancer cells in the metastatic foci mostly show epithelial appearances, suggesting MET also takes place in cancers. Whether or not the EMT/MET process in cancers utilizes a similar transcriptional program as in normal development is not fully clear. It is conceivable that rather than EMT itself, but the acquisition of plasticity to freely undergo both EMT/MET may be a more important characteristic of cancer stem cells as well as normal stem cells.

GLYCANS ASSOCIATED WITH HUMAN EMBRYONIC STEM CELLS AND CANCER STEM CELLS

Appearance of Classical Human Embryonic Stem Cell Marker Glycans, SSEA-3/-4, in Cancer Stem Cells

Cell surface glycans are known to be good markers for embryonic stem (ES) cells in the field of stem cell research. The first example is SSEA-1, which appears in the early stages of murine preimplantation embryos in a stage-specific manner [83]. However, SSEA-1 is not considered to be a good ES cell marker in humans, because it appears at much later stages of embryonic development compared to mice. Instead, SSEA-3 and SSEA-4 glycans are regarded as good markers for human ES cells [84]. They both appear not only in embryonic stem cells, but also in iPS cells. These glycans were utilized in discriminating the true iPS cell colonies out of many other colonies when human iPS cells were first generated by transfection of OCT3/4, SOX2, KLF4, and c-MYC [54].

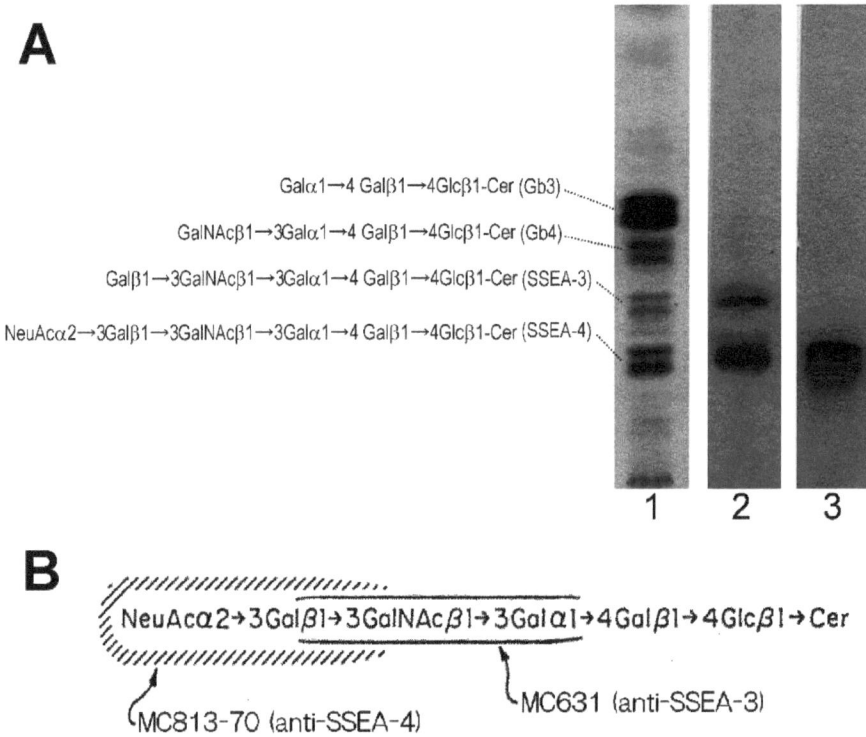

Fig. (7). Total glycan structures of SSEA-3 and SSEA-4 glycolipids and reactivity of specific antibodies. Panel **A**, structures of SSEA-3, SSEA-4 and related glycolipids and the results of TLC-immunostaining with the specific antibodies. In TLC staining, lane 1; total glycolipids of human EC cells 2102Ep, lanes 2 and 3, immunostaining of the same glycolipid samples with the antibodies MC631 (anti-SSEA-3) and MC813-70 (anti-SSEA-4), respectively. Panel **B**, a scheme for the glycan epitopes recognized by these antibodies. (Adapted from reference [84]).

SSEA-3/-4 glycans are classified into the globo-series glycolipids [84], which compose a unique series of glycolipids having glycan structures confined to glycolipids, and are not easily detectable in glycoproteins. Nowadays SSEA-3 usually refers to a non-sialylated globoseries glycolipid having five sugar residues (Gb5), while SSEA-4 refers to the sialylated Gb5. It is notable that the antibody directed to SSEA-3 (MC631) actually reacted to both Gb5 and sialylated Gb5, suggesting that the antibody recognizes an internal epitope shared with both glycolipids (Fig. **7**), while the antibody directed to SSEA-4 (MC813-70) seemed to recognize a terminal epitope carried by the glycan, and reacted only with sialylated Gb5 but not with non-sialylated Gb5. After elucidation of total structures of antigenic glycolipids [84], the term SSEA-3 was re-defined and confined to Gb5, because it was not convenient to define two different glycolipids by a single term "SSEA-3." This must be noted when researchers perform studies using the antibodies; for instance, theoretically there should be no such phenotype as SSEA-3(-)/SSEA-4(+), as far as these antibodies are used as the tools for detection.

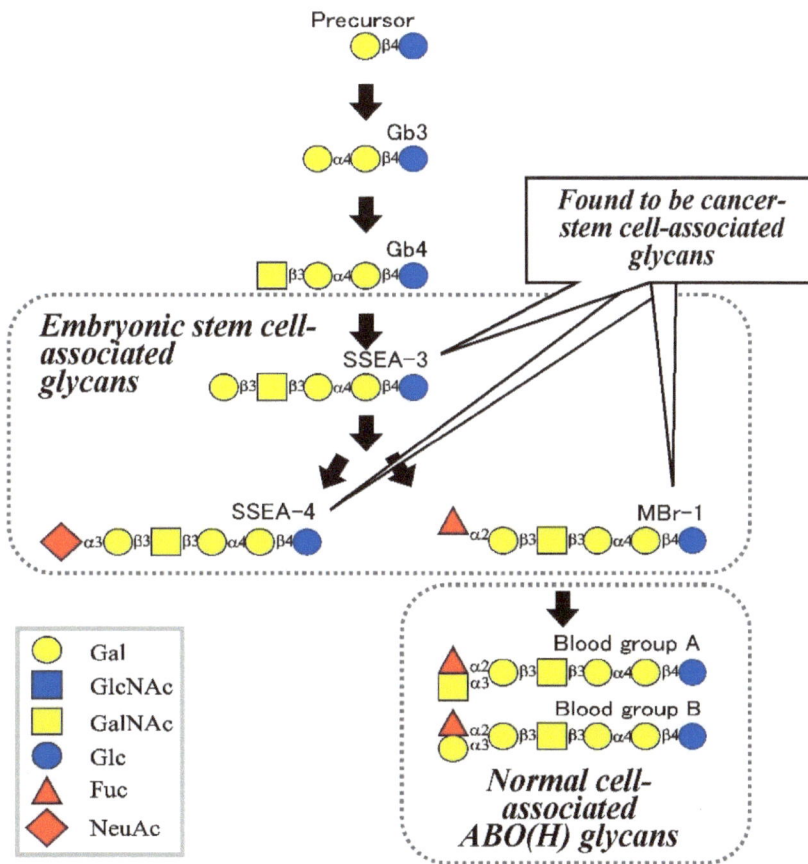

Fig. (8). Biosynthetic pathway for globoseries glycolipids including SSEA-3 and SSEA-4 also contains cancer-stem cell-associated glycans.

The synthetic pathway for these glycans is shown in Fig. (**8**). Further studies on the globoseries glycolipids indicated that SSEA-3 is further modified at the terminus by fucose through α1-2 linkage, forming O(H)-type structure in the ABO blood group system in some tissues, and the glycolipid was called Globo-H [85, 86]. This is eventually modified further by GalNAc through α 1-3 linkage, forming a blood group A-type structure [87]. A glycolipid having the glycan structure of disialylated SSEA-3 was also identified [88]. Even the glycolipid having the SSEA-1 structure linked to the terminus of SSEA-3 glycolipid was detected in murine kidney [89, 90].

Among these extended globoseries glycolipids described above, right now only SSEA-3, SSEA-4 and Globo-H are known to be preferentially expressed on human embryonic stem cells. These three classical glycans are known to be expressed also in human cancers (Fig. **8**). There had been sporadic publications reporting that SSEA-3/-4 glycans sometimes appear in human cancer cells [91 - 94], and it was recently reported that these glycans are specifically expressed in cancer stem-like cells [95, 96]. It is interesting to note that the glycan markers initially described to be specific to embryonic stem cells started to be recognized also as markers for cancer stem cells. This would suggest the presence of a common induction mechanism for these glycans shared by embryonic stem cells and cancer stem cells. Globo-H is exceptional in that this glycolipid was initially described to be specifically expressed in breast cancers, and later found to be expressed in embryonic stem cells.

SSEA-1 glycan, which is usually not regarded as a human embryonic stem cell marker, appears in human neural stem cells in the subventricular zone, and is supposed to be a good marker for these cells. SSEA-1 is found to be preferentially expressed in cancer stem cells of human gliomas [97 - 99] in addition to murine brain tumors [99, 100]. Although rather tissue-specific, this can be regarded as an additional example indicating the close relationship of glycans expressed in normal stem cells and cancer stem cells.

More than 30 years have elapsed since the discovery of SSEA-3 and SSEA-4 glycans, but the mechanisms of how these glycans appear specifically on the surface of ES cells have not been elucidated yet. It is well-known that a combination of several transcription factors such as OCT3/4, Nanog and Sox-2 play critical roles in maintaining the stemness in these cells [54], while transcriptional regulation of ES cell-associated glycan expression still remains largely unknown.

Lactoseries Glycans Recently Emerging as Human Embryonic and Cancer Stem Cell Markers

TRA-1-60 is an embryonic stem cell-specific glycan, which is defined by a monoclonal antibody generated at the same period as anti-SSEA-3 and SSEA-4 antibodies [101, 102]. This glycan was also applied for identifying the iPS cell colonies when the first human iPS cells were established as well as SSEA-3 and SSEA-4 [54]. The glycan has long been assumed to have a keratan sulfate-like structure modified by sialic acid and sulfate residues [103]. However, recently the TRA-1-60 glycan was reported to be a type 1 chain lactosamine glycan, having common backbone structures with glycans carried by both glycolipids and glycoproteins, having no sialic acid/sulfate modification at least at their antigenic epitope [104]. This indicated that the reactivity of anti-TRA-1-60 is very similar to that of K21 antibody previously raised against Tera-1, a human teratocarcinoma cell line. K21 reacted with glycans having a type 1 chain lactosamine structure [105], which was later confirmed to recognize the Lc_4 glycolipid, which belongs to the lactoseries glycolipid group but not to the globoseries glycolipids [106]. The recently-introduced fucosylated stem cell-associated glycan, SSEA-5, is a type 1 chain H(O) antigen, which again has the backbone structure of the type-1 chain lactosamine glycan [107].

The synthetic pathway for these glycans is shown in Fig. (**9**). The TRA-1-60, K21 and SSEA-5 glycans belong to the same group of glycans and share the same enzymes in most steps of their synthetic pathways, while their synthetic pathway is independent from that for the synthesis of globo-series glycolipids. These findings indicate that there is a distinct group of glycans specific to human embryonic stem cells, which is structurally and metabolically different from a group of globoseries glycolipids such as SSEA-3/-4 and Globo-H.

Finally, sialyl Lewis A, another type 1 chain lactosamine glycan, was shown to behave as a glycan marker for human embryonic stem cells; it is expressed in human ES cells, and disappears upon ES cell differentiation [107]. Sialyl Lewis A is the well-known cancer-associated glycan, and we reported significant induction of sialyl Lewis A in cancer stem-like cells derived from EMT of cultured colon cancer cells [76]. These findings again strongly suggest that there are some common features between glycans specific to ES cells and those associated with cancer stem cells. The TRA-1-60, SSEA-5 and sialyl Lewis A glycans are structurally closely related, and share the same enzymes in most steps of their synthetic pathway, which is the synthetic pathway for type 1 chain lactosamine glycans (Fig. **9**).

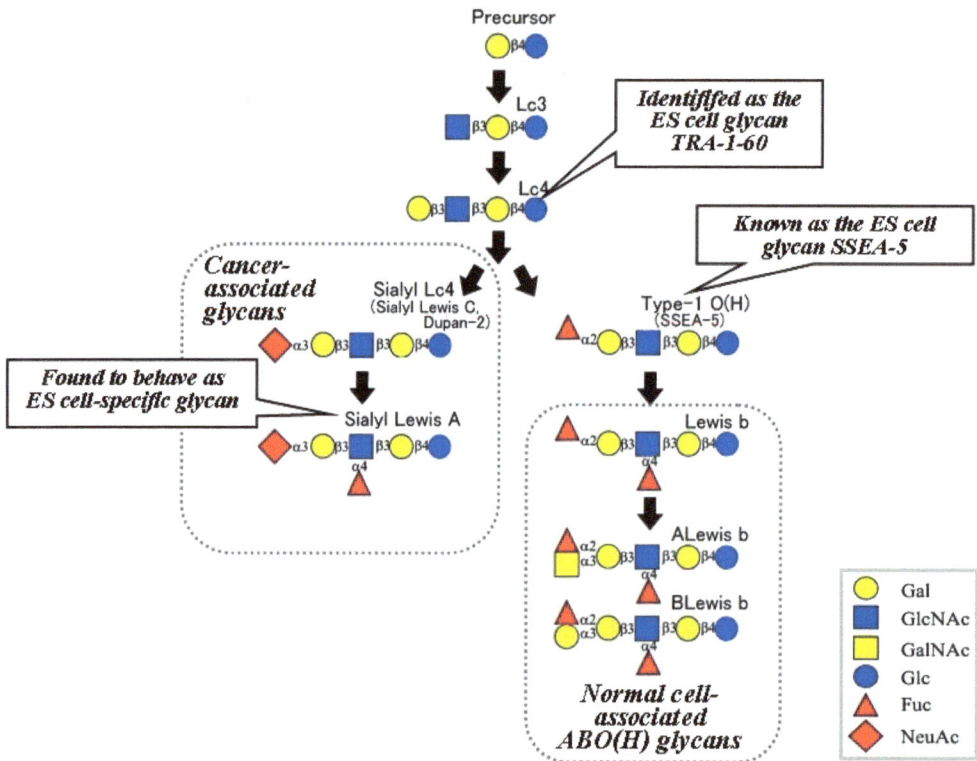

Fig. (9). Biosynthetic pathway for type-1-chain lactosamine glycans contains classical cancer-associated glycans and several recently-emerging embryonic stem-cell specific glycans.

The same synthetic pathway contains sialylated type 1 chain lactosamine (sialyl Lc4, or sialyl Lewis C), which is another cancer-associated glycan, Dupan-2, a marker for pancreas cancers (Fig. **9**) [108]. It is conceivable that this glycan may also behave as an embryonic stem cell marker, as the K4 antibody recognizing this glycan [106] is known to be preferentially expressed in human teratocarcinoma cells [105].

The type 1 chain lactosamine glycans contain important cancer-associated glycans such as sialyl Lewis A, and have been vigorously studied mainly by researchers in the oncology field for more than 30 years. Quite recently, these glycans were found to behave as embryonic stem cell markers in the field of embryology. On the other hand, SSEA-3 and SSEA-4 are very classical embryonic stem cell markers, and also have a more than 30 year history of investigation in the field of embryology. It is only recently that these glycans began to be recognized as markers of cancer stem cells in the oncology field.

CONCLUSION

Cell surface glycans undergo drastic changes during malignant transformation, and the glycans which preferentially appear in cancers are clinically utilized as diagnostic markers for human cancers. Such tumor marker glycans include sialyl Lewis A, sialyl Lewis X, Dupan-2 and sialyl Tn, expression of some of which is known to be enhanced in so-called cancer stem cells. On the other hand, cell surface glycans are also known to be good markers for human pluripotent embryonic stem cells. Typical glycan markers for human embryonic stem cells include SSEA-3, SSEA-4, TRA-1-60 and SSEA-5. The classical human embryonic stem cell markers such as SSEA-3 and SSEA-4 belong to a group of glycans called globoseries glycolipids. This group of glycans also include a glycan marker for breast cancer, Globo-H. These globoseries glycans are recently known to be frequently expressed in human cancers, especially in cancer stem cells. Recently another group of glycans are emerging as markers for human embryonic stem cells, which is type 1 chain lactosamine (lactoseries) glycans, including TRA-1-60 and SSEA-5. This group also includes typical glycan markers for cancers, such as sialyl Lewis A and Dupan-2. Recently sialyl Lewis A was shown to be expressed in human embryonic stem cells, and behaves as an embryonic stem-cell specific marker. Thus, a glycan initially described as cancer-associated is now known to be an embryonic stem cell marker, while glycans formerly regarded to be typical embryonic stem cell markers are now shown to be cancer stem cell markers. The field of study of cancer stem cell glycans is thus almost going to merge with the field of study for embryonic stem cell glycans. This suggests the presence of a common induction mechanism for these glycans shared by embryonic stem cells and cancer stem cells. Transcription factors such as OCT3/4, Nanog and Sox2 are recognized to play critical roles in maintaining the stemness in both embryonic and cancer stem cells. However, the regulatory mechanisms for stem-cell specific glycan expression remains largely unknown. At present, glycan-related genes responsible for synthesis of the stem-cell specific glycans are known to be regulated through epigenetic modification, by microenvironmental factors such as hypoxia, and during the biological process like epithelial-mesenchymal transition.

CONFLICT OF INTEREST

The authors confirm that they have no conflict of interest to declare for this publication.

ACKNOWLEDGEMENTS

This work was supported in part by a grant-in-aid from the Ministry of Science and Technology [104-2314-B-001-001, and 104-2314-B-001-006], and a grant from Academia Sinica and Ministry of Science and Technology, Taiwan [104-0210-01-09-03].

REFERENCES

[1]   Kannagi R, Kitahara A, Itai S, *et al.* Quantitative and qualitative characterization of human cancer-associated serum glycoprotein antigens expressing epitopes consisting of sialyl or sialyl-fucosyl type 1 chain. Cancer Res 1988; 48(13): 3856-63.
        [PMID: 2454154]

[2]   Itai S, Arii S, Tobe R, *et al.* Significance of 2-3 and 2-6 sialylation of Lewis a antigen in pancreas cancer. Cancer 1988; 61(4): 775-87.
        [http://dx.doi.org/10.1002/1097-0142(19880215)61:4<775::AID-CNCR2820610423>3.0.CO;2-U]
        [PMID: 3422178]

[3]   Itai S, Nishikata J, Yoneda T, *et al.* Tissue distribution of sialyl 2-3 and 2-6 Lewis a antigens and the significance of serum 2-3/2-6 sialyl Lewis a antigen ratio for the differential diagnosis of malignant and benign disorders of the digestive tract. Cancer 1991; 67: 1576-87.
        [http://dx.doi.org/10.1002/1097-0142(19910315)67:6<1576::AID-CNCR2820670620>3.0.CO;2-2]
        [PMID: 2001547]

[4] Kannagi R. Carbohydrate antigen sialyl Lewis a--its pathophysiological significance and induction mechanism in cancer progression. Chang Gung Med J 2007; 30(3): 189-209.
[PMID: 17760270]

[5] Izawa M, Kumamoto K, Mitsuoka C, *et al.* Expression of sialyl 6-sulfo Lewis X is inversely correlated with conventional sialyl Lewis X expression in human colorectal cancer. Cancer Res 2000; 60(5): 1410-6.
[PMID: 10728707]

[6] Miyazaki K, Ohmori K, Izawa M, *et al.* Loss of disialyl Lewis[a], the ligand for lymphocyte inhibitory receptor Siglec-7, associated with increased sialyl Lewis[a] expression on human colon cancers. Cancer Res 2004; 64: 4498-505.
[http://dx.doi.org/10.1158/0008-5472.CAN-03-3614] [PMID: 15231659]

[7] Lim K-T, Miyazaki K, Kimura N, Izawa M, Kannagi R. Clinical application of functional glycoproteomics - dissection of glycotopes carried by soluble CD44 variants in sera of patients with cancers. Proteomics 2008; 8(16): 3263-73.
[http://dx.doi.org/10.1002/pmic.200800147] [PMID: 18690645]

[8] Bowden NA, Croft A, Scott RJ. Gene expression profiling in familial adenomatous polyposis adenomas and desmoid disease. Hered Cancer Clin Pract 2007; 5(2): 79-96.
[http://dx.doi.org/10.1186/1897-4287-5-2-79] [PMID: 19725988]

[9] Young WW Jr, Mills SE, Lippert MC, Ahmed P, Lau SK. Deletion of antigens of the Lewis a/b blood group family in human prostatic carcinoma. Am J Pathol 1988; 131(3): 578-86.
[PMID: 2454582]

[10] Potapenko IO, Haakensen VD, Lüders T, *et al.* Glycan gene expression signatures in normal and malignant breast tissue; possible role in diagnosis and progression. Mol Oncol 2010; 4(2): 98-118.
[http://dx.doi.org/10.1016/j.molonc.2009.12.001] [PMID: 20060370]

[11] Senda M, Ito A, Tsuchida A, *et al.* Identification and expression of a sialyltransferase responsible for the synthesis of disialylgalactosylgloboside in normal and malignant kidney cells: downregulation of ST6GalNAc VI in renal cancers. Biochem J 2007; 402(3): 459-70.
[http://dx.doi.org/10.1042/BJ20061118] [PMID: 17123352]

[12] Kroes RA, Dawson G, Moskal JR. Focused microarray analysis of glyco-gene expression in human glioblastomas. J Neurochem 2007; 103 (Suppl. 1): 14-24.
[http://dx.doi.org/10.1111/j.1471-4159.2007.04780.x] [PMID: 17986135]

[13] Shamsuddin AK, Weiss L, Phelps PC, Trump BF. Colon epithelium. IV. Human colon carcinogenesis. Changes in human colon mucosa adjacent to and remote from carcinomas of the colon. J Natl Cancer Inst 1981; 66(2): 413-9.
[PMID: 6935488]

[14] Yusa A, Miyazaki K, Kimura N, Izawa M, Kannagi R. Epigenetic silencing of the sulfate transporter gene *DTDST* induces sialyl Lewis[x] expression and accelerates proliferation of colon cancer cells. Cancer Res 2010; 70(10): 4064-73.
[http://dx.doi.org/10.1158/0008-5472.CAN-09-2383] [PMID: 20460514]

[15] Lee S, Bang S, Song K, Lee I. Differential expression in normal-adenoma-carcinoma sequence

suggests complex molecular carcinogenesis in colon. Oncol Rep 2006; 16(4): 747-54.
[PMID: 16969489]

[16]   Miyazaki K, Sakuma K, Kawamura YI, *et al.* Colonic epithelial cells express specific ligands for mucosal macrophage immunosuppressive receptors siglec-7 and -9. J Immunol 2012; 188(9): 4690-700.
[http://dx.doi.org/10.4049/jimmunol.1100605] [PMID: 22467657]

[17]   Oshima M, Dinchuk JE, Kargman SL, *et al.* Suppression of intestinal polyposis in Apc delta716 knockout mice by inhibition of cyclooxygenase 2 (COX-2). Cell 1996; 87(5): 803-9.
[http://dx.doi.org/10.1016/S0092-8674(00)81988-1] [PMID: 8945508]

[18]   Kominato Y, Hata Y, Takizawa H, Tsuchiya T, Tsukada J, Yamamoto F. Expression of human histo-blood group ABO genes is dependent upon DNA methylation of the promoter region. J Biol Chem 1999; 274(52): 37240-50.
[http://dx.doi.org/10.1074/jbc.274.52.37240] [PMID: 10601288]

[19]   Chihara Y, Sugano K, Kobayashi A, *et al.* Loss of blood group A antigen expression in bladder cancer caused by allelic loss and/or methylation of the ABO gene. Lab Invest 2005; 85(7): 895-907.
[http://dx.doi.org/10.1038/labinvest.3700268] [PMID: 15880137]

[20]   Kawamura YI, Toyota M, Kawashima R, *et al.* DNA hypermethylation contributes to incomplete synthesis of carbohydrate determinants in gastrointestinal cancer. Gastroenterology 2008; 135(1): 142-151.e3.
[http://dx.doi.org/10.1053/j.gastro.2008.03.031] [PMID: 18485915]

[21]   Kannagi R, Izawa M, Koike T, Miyazaki K, Kimura N. Carbohydrate-mediated cell adhesion in cancer metastasis and angiogenesis. Cancer Sci 2004; 95(5): 377-84.
[http://dx.doi.org/10.1111/j.1349-7006.2004.tb03219.x] [PMID: 15132763]

[22]   Kannagi R, Yin J, Miyazaki K, Izawa M. Current relevance of incomplete synthesis and neo-synthesis for cancer-associated alteration of carbohydrate determinants-Hakomori's concepts revisited. Biochim Biophys Acta 2008; 1780: 525-31.

[23]   Miyamoto K, Asada K, Fukutomi T, *et al.* Methylation-associated silencing of heparan sulfate D-glucosaminyl 3-O-sulfotransferase-2 (3-OST-2) in human breast, colon, lung and pancreatic cancers. Oncogene 2003; 22(2): 274-80.
[http://dx.doi.org/10.1038/sj.onc.1206146] [PMID: 12527896]

[24]   Hwang JA, Kim Y, Hong SH, *et al.* Epigenetic inactivation of heparan sulfate (glucosamine) 3--sulfotransferase 2 in lung cancer and its role in tumorigenesis. PLoS One 2013; 8(11): e79634.
[http://dx.doi.org/10.1371/journal.pone.0079634] [PMID: 24265783]

[25]   Fuster MM, Esko JD. The sweet and sour of cancer: glycans as novel therapeutic targets. Nat Rev Cancer 2005; 5(7): 526-42.
[http://dx.doi.org/10.1038/nrc1649] [PMID: 16069816]

[26]   Zhang L, Shi J, Ji M, *et al.* Methylation analysis of drug metabolism and transport genes in papillary thyroid cancer. Adv Sci Lett 2012; 17: 243-50.
[http://dx.doi.org/10.1166/asl.2012.4245]

[27]   Fussbroich B, Wagener N, Macher-Goeppinger S, *et al.* EZH2 depletion blocks the proliferation of

colon cancer cells. PLoS One 2011; 6(7): e21651.
[http://dx.doi.org/10.1371/journal.pone.0021651] [PMID: 21765901]

[28]   Hahn MA, Li AX, Wu X, *et al.* Loss of the polycomb mark from bivalent promoters leads to activation of cancer-promoting genes in colorectal tumors. Cancer Res 2014; 74(13): 3617-29.
[http://dx.doi.org/10.1158/0008-5472.CAN-13-3147] [PMID: 24786786]

[29]   Hakomori S, Kannagi R. Glycosphingolipids as tumor-associated and differentiation markers. J Natl Cancer Inst 1983; 71(2): 231-51.
[PMID: 6576183]

[30]   Kannagi R, Sakuma K, Miyazaki K, *et al.* Altered expression of glycan genes in cancers induced by epigenetic silencing and tumor hypoxia: clues in the ongoing search for new tumor markers. Cancer Sci 2010; 101(3): 586-93.
[http://dx.doi.org/10.1111/j.1349-7006.2009.01455.x] [PMID: 20085584]

[31]   Campbell F, Appleton MA, Fuller CE, *et al.* Racial variation in the O-acetylation phenotype of human colonic mucosa. J Pathol 1994; 174(3): 169-74.
[http://dx.doi.org/10.1002/path.1711740305] [PMID: 7823249]

[32]   Okayasu I, Hana K, Tsuruta T, *et al.* Significant increase of colonic mutated crypts correlates with age in sporadic cancer and diverticulosis cases, with higher frequency in the left- than right-sided colorectum. Cancer Sci 2006; 97(5): 362-7.
[http://dx.doi.org/10.1111/j.1349-7006.2006.00181.x] [PMID: 16630132]

[33]   O'Carroll D, Erhardt S, Pagani M, Barton SC, Surani MA, Jenuwein T. The polycomb-group gene Ezh2 is required for early mouse development. Mol Cell Biol 2001; 21(13): 4330-6.
[http://dx.doi.org/10.1128/MCB.21.13.4330-4336.2001] [PMID: 11390661]

[34]   Mikkelsen TS, Ku M, Jaffe DB, *et al.* Genome-wide maps of chromatin state in pluripotent and lineage-committed cells. Nature 2007; 448(7153): 553-60.
[http://dx.doi.org/10.1038/nature06008] [PMID: 17603471]

[35]   Chen T, Dent SY. Chromatin modifiers and remodellers: regulators of cellular differentiation. Nat Rev Genet 2014; 15(2): 93-106.
[http://dx.doi.org/10.1038/nrg3607] [PMID: 24366184]

[36]   Ravillah D, Mohammed A, Qian L, *et al.* Chemopreventive effects of an HDAC2-selective inhibitor on rat colon carcinogenesis and APCmin/+ mouse intestinal tumorigenesis. J Pharmacol Exp Ther 2014; 348(1): 59-68.
[http://dx.doi.org/10.1124/jpet.113.208645] [PMID: 24218540]

[37]   Timp W, Feinberg AP. Cancer as a dysregulated epigenome allowing cellular growth advantage at the expense of the host. Nat Rev Cancer 2013; 13(7): 497-510.
[http://dx.doi.org/10.1038/nrc3486] [PMID: 23760024]

[38]   Chu CS, Lo PW, Yeh YH, *et al.* O-GlcNAcylation regulates EZH2 protein stability and function. Proc Natl Acad Sci USA 2014; 111(4): 1355-60.
[http://dx.doi.org/10.1073/pnas.1323226111] [PMID: 24474760]

[39]   Kannagi R. Molecular mechanism for cancer-associated induction of sialyl Lewis X and sialyl Lewis A expression-The Warburg effect revisited. Glycoconj J 2004; 20(5): 353-64.

[http://dx.doi.org/10.1023/B:GLYC.0000033631.35357.41] [PMID: 15229399]

[40]   Koike T, Kimura N, Miyazaki K, *et al.* Hypoxia induces adhesion molecules on cancer cells: A missing link between Warburg effect and induction of selectin-ligand carbohydrates. Proc Natl Acad Sci USA 2004; 101(21): 8132-7.
[http://dx.doi.org/10.1073/pnas.0402088101] [PMID: 15141079]

[41]   Tei K, Kawakami-Kimura N, Taguchi O, *et al.* Roles of cell adhesion molecules in tumor angiogenesis induced by cotransplantation of cancer and endothelial cells to nude rats. Cancer Res 2002; 62(21): 6289-96.
[PMID: 12414659]

[42]   Yin J, Miyazaki K, Shaner RL, Merrill AH Jr, Kannagi R. Altered sphingolipid metabolism induced by tumor hypoxia - new vistas in glycolipid tumor markers. FEBS Lett 2010; 584(9): 1872-8.
[http://dx.doi.org/10.1016/j.febslet.2009.11.019] [PMID: 19913543]

[43]   Tanaka K, Tamiya-Koizumi K, Yamada M, Murate T, Kannagi R, Kyogashima M. Individual profiles of free ceramide species and the constituent ceramide species of sphingomyelin and neutral glycosphingolipid and their alteration according to the sequential changes of environmental oxygen content in human colorectal cancer Caco-2 cells. Glycoconj J 2014; 31(3): 209-19.
[http://dx.doi.org/10.1007/s10719-013-9511-9] [PMID: 24310545]

[44]   Yin J, Hashimoto A, Izawa M, *et al.* Hypoxic culture induces expression of sialin, a sialic acid transporter, and cancer-associated gangliosides containing non-human sialic acid on human cancer cells. Cancer Res 2006; 66(6): 2937-45.
[http://dx.doi.org/10.1158/0008-5472.CAN-05-2615] [PMID: 16540641]

[45]   Go S, Sato C, Yin J, Kannagi R, Kitajima K. Hypoxia-enhanced expression of free deaminoneuraminic acid in human cancer cells. Biochem Biophys Res Commun 2007; 357(2): 537-42.
[http://dx.doi.org/10.1016/j.bbrc.2007.03.181] [PMID: 17434449]

[46]   Inoue S, Sato C, Kitajima K. Extensive enrichment of N-glycolylneuraminic acid in extracellular sialoglycoproteins abundantly synthesized and secreted by human cancer cells. Glycobiology 2010; 20(6): 752-62.
[http://dx.doi.org/10.1093/glycob/cwq030] [PMID: 20197272]

[47]   Närvä E, Pursiheimo JP, Laiho A, *et al.* Continuous hypoxic culturing of human embryonic stem cells enhances SSEA-3 and MYC levels. PLoS One 2013; 8(11): e78847.
[http://dx.doi.org/10.1371/journal.pone.0078847] [PMID: 24236059]

[48]   Ezashi T, Das P, Roberts RM. Low O2 tensions and the prevention of differentiation of hES cells. Proc Natl Acad Sci USA 2005; 102(13): 4783-8.
[http://dx.doi.org/10.1073/pnas.0501283102] [PMID: 15772165]

[49]   Simon MC, Keith B. The role of oxygen availability in embryonic development and stem cell function. Nat Rev Mol Cell Biol 2008; 9(4): 285-96.
[http://dx.doi.org/10.1038/nrm2354] [PMID: 18285802]

[50]   Covello KL, Kehler J, Yu H, *et al.* HIF-2α regulates Oct-4: effects of hypoxia on stem cell function, embryonic development, and tumor growth. Genes Dev 2006; 20(5): 557-70.
[http://dx.doi.org/10.1101/gad.1399906] [PMID: 16510872]

[51]   Gordan JD, Bertout JA, Hu CJ, Diehl JA, Simon MC. HIF-2α promotes hypoxic cell proliferation by enhancing c-myc transcriptional activity. Cancer Cell 2007; 11(4): 335-47.
[http://dx.doi.org/10.1016/j.ccr.2007.02.006] [PMID: 17418410]

[52]   Petruzzelli R, Christensen DR, Parry KL, Sanchez-Elsner T, Houghton FD. HIF-2α regulates NANOG expression in human embryonic stem cells following hypoxia and reoxygenation through the interaction with an Oct-Sox cis regulatory element. PLoS One 2014; 9(10): e108309.
[http://dx.doi.org/10.1371/journal.pone.0108309] [PMID: 25271810]

[53]   Takahashi K, Yamanaka S. Induction of pluripotent stem cells from mouse embryonic and adult fibroblast cultures by defined factors. Cell 2006; 126(4): 663-76.
[http://dx.doi.org/10.1016/j.cell.2006.07.024] [PMID: 16904174]

[54]   Takahashi K, Tanabe K, Ohnuki M, *et al.* Induction of pluripotent stem cells from adult human fibroblasts by defined factors. Cell 2007; 131(5): 861-72.
[http://dx.doi.org/10.1016/j.cell.2007.11.019] [PMID: 18035408]

[55]   Yoshida Y, Takahashi K, Okita K, Ichisaka T, Yamanaka S. Hypoxia enhances the generation of induced pluripotent stem cells. Cell Stem Cell 2009; 5(3): 237-41.
[http://dx.doi.org/10.1016/j.stem.2009.08.001] [PMID: 19716359]

[56]   Nombela-Arrieta C, Silberstein LE. The science behind the hypoxic niche of hematopoietic stem and progenitors. Hematology Am Soc Hematol Educ Program 2014; 2014(1): 542-7.
[http://dx.doi.org/10.1182/asheducation-2014.1.542]

[57]   Jež M, Rožman P, Ivanović Z, Bas T. Concise review: the role of oxygen in hematopoietic stem cell physiology. J Cell Physiol 2015; 230(9): 1999-2005.
[http://dx.doi.org/10.1002/jcp.24953] [PMID: 25655806]

[58]   Tan SC, Gomes RS, Yeoh KK, *et al.* Preconditioning of cardiosphere-derived cells with hypoxia or prolyl-4-hydroxylase inhibitors increases stemness and decreases reliance on oxidative metabolism. Cell Transplant 2015. [Epub ahead of print].
[PMID: 25751158]

[59]   Li L, Candelario KM, Thomas K, *et al.* Hypoxia inducible factor-1α (HIF-1α) is required for neural stem cell maintenance and vascular stability in the adult mouse SVZ. J Neurosci 2014; 34(50): 16713-9.
[http://dx.doi.org/10.1523/JNEUROSCI.4590-13.2014] [PMID: 25505323]

[60]   Hoch AI, Leach JK. Concise review: optimizing expansion of bone marrow mesenchymal stem/stromal cells for clinical applications. Stem Cells Transl Med 2014; 3(5): 643-52.
[http://dx.doi.org/10.5966/sctm.2013-0196] [PMID: 24682286]

[61]   Choi JR, Pingguan-Murphy B, Wan Abas WA, *et al.* Impact of low oxygen tension on stemness, proliferation and differentiation potential of human adipose-derived stem cells. Biochem Biophys Res Commun 2014; 448(2): 218-24.
[http://dx.doi.org/10.1016/j.bbrc.2014.04.096] [PMID: 24785372]

[62]   Jarecki J, Johnson E, Krasnow MA. Oxygen regulation of airway branching in Drosophila is mediated by branchless FGF. Cell 1999; 99(2): 211-20.
[http://dx.doi.org/10.1016/S0092-8674(00)81652-9] [PMID: 10535739]

[63]   van Tuyl M, Liu J, Wang J, Kuliszewski M, Tibboel D, Post M. Role of oxygen and vascular development in epithelial branching morphogenesis of the developing mouse lung. Am J Physiol Lung Cell Mol Physiol 2005; 288(1): L167-78.
[http://dx.doi.org/10.1152/ajplung.00185.2004] [PMID: 15377493]

[64]   Gebb SA, Fox K, Vaughn J, McKean D, Jones PL. Fetal oxygen tension promotes tenascin--dependent lung branching morphogenesis. Dev Dyn 2005; 234(1): 1-10.
[http://dx.doi.org/10.1002/dvdy.20500] [PMID: 16086306]

[65]   Gebb SA, Jones PL. Hypoxia and lung branching morphogenesis. Adv Exp Med Biol 2003; 543: 117-25.
[http://dx.doi.org/10.1007/978-1-4419-8997-0_8] [PMID: 14713117]

[66]   Pimton P, Lecht S, Stabler CT, Johannes G, Schulman ES, Lelkes PI. Hypoxia enhances differentiation of mouse embryonic stem cells into definitive endoderm and distal lung cells. Stem Cells Dev 2015; 24(5): 663-76.
[http://dx.doi.org/10.1089/scd.2014.0343] [PMID: 25226206]

[67]   Miyake M, Zenita K, Tanaka O, Okada Y, Kannagi R. Stage-specific expression of SSEA-1-related antigens in the developing lung of human embryos and its relation to the distribution of these antigens in lung cancers. Cancer Res 1988; 48(24 Pt 1): 7150-8.
[PMID: 2903794]

[68]   Itai S, Nishikata J, Takahashi N, *et al.* Differentiation-dependent expression of I and sialyl I antigens in the developing lung of human embryos and in lung cancers. Cancer Res 1990; 50(23): 7603-11.
[PMID: 1979246]

[69]   Compernolle V, Brusselmans K, Acker T, *et al.* Loss of HIF-2α and inhibition of VEGF impair fetal lung maturation, whereas treatment with VEGF prevents fatal respiratory distress in premature mice. Nat Med 2002; 8(7): 702-10.
[PMID: 12053176]

[70]   Tsuji K, Kitamura S, Makino H. Hypoxia-inducible factor 1α regulates branching morphogenesis during kidney development. Biochem Biophys Res Commun 2014; 447(1): 108-14.
[http://dx.doi.org/10.1016/j.bbrc.2014.03.111] [PMID: 24690177]

[71]   Ricci-Vitiani L, Fabrizi E, Palio E, De Maria R. Colon cancer stem cells. J Mol Med 2009; 87(11): 1097-104.
[http://dx.doi.org/10.1007/s00109-009-0518-4] [PMID: 19727638]

[72]   Boman BM, Wicha MS. Cancer stem cells: a step toward the cure. J Clin Oncol 2008; 26(17): 2795-9.
[http://dx.doi.org/10.1200/JCO.2008.17.7436] [PMID: 18539956]

[73]   Mani SA, Guo W, Liao MJ, *et al.* The epithelial-mesenchymal transition generates cells with properties of stem cells. Cell 2008; 133(4): 704-15.
[http://dx.doi.org/10.1016/j.cell.2008.03.027] [PMID: 18485877]

[74]   Guan F, Handa K, Hakomori SI. Specific glycosphingolipids mediate epithelial-to-mesenchymal transition of human and mouse epithelial cell lines. Proc Natl Acad Sci USA 2009; 106(18): 7461-6.
[http://dx.doi.org/10.1073/pnas.0902368106] [PMID: 19380734]

[75]   Guan F, Schaffer L, Handa K, Hakomori SI. Functional role of gangliotetraosylceramide in epithelial-

to-mesenchymal transition process induced by hypoxia and by TGF-β. FASEB J 2010; 24(12): 4889-903.
[http://dx.doi.org/10.1096/fj.10-162107] [PMID: 20720159]

[76]   Sakuma K, Aoki M, Kannagi R. Transcription factors c-Myc and CDX2 mediate E-selectin ligand expression in colon cancer cells undergoing EGF/bFGF-induced epithelial-mesenchymal transition. Proc Natl Acad Sci USA 2012; 109(20): 7776-81.
[http://dx.doi.org/10.1073/pnas.1111135109] [PMID: 22547830]

[77]   Ono M, Sakamoto M, Ino Y, *et al.* Cancer cell morphology at the invasive front and expression of cell adhesion-related carbohydrate in the primary lesion of patients with colorectal carcinoma with liver metastasis. Cancer 1996; 78(6): 1179-86.
[http://dx.doi.org/10.1002/(SICI)1097-0142(19960915)78:6<1179::AID-CNCR3>3.0.CO;2-5] [PMID: 8826938]

[78]   Phillips ML, Nudelman E, Gaeta FC, *et al.* ELAM-1 mediates cell adhesion by recognition of a carbohydrate ligand, sialyl-Le^x. Science 1990; 250(4984): 1130-2.
[http://dx.doi.org/10.1126/science.1701274] [PMID: 1701274]

[79]   Takada A, Ohmori K, Takahashi N, *et al.* Adhesion of human cancer cells to vascular endothelium mediated by a carbohydrate antigen, sialyl Lewis A. Biochem Biophys Res Commun 1991; 179(2): 713-9.
[http://dx.doi.org/10.1016/0006-291X(91)91875-D] [PMID: 1716885]

[80]   Takada A, Ohmori K, Yoneda T, *et al.* Contribution of carbohydrate antigens sialyl Lewis A and sialyl Lewis X to adhesion of human cancer cells to vascular endothelium. Cancer Res 1993; 53(2): 354-61.
[PMID: 7678075]

[81]   Acloque H, Adams MS, Fishwick K, Bronner-Fraser M, Nieto MA. Epithelial-mesenchymal transitions: the importance of changing cell state in development and disease. J Clin Invest 2009; 119(6): 1438-49.
[http://dx.doi.org/10.1172/JCI38019] [PMID: 19487820]

[82]   Kalluri R, Weinberg RA. The basics of epithelial-mesenchymal transition. J Clin Invest 2009; 119(6): 1420-8.
[http://dx.doi.org/10.1172/JCI39104] [PMID: 19487818]

[83]   Solter D, Knowles BB. Monoclonal antibody defining a stage-specific mouse embryonic antigen (SSEA-1). Proc Natl Acad Sci USA 1978; 75(11): 5565-9.
[http://dx.doi.org/10.1073/pnas.75.11.5565] [PMID: 281705]

[84]   Kannagi R, Cochran NA, Ishigami F, *et al.* Stage-specific embryonic antigens (SSEA-3 and -4) are epitopes of a unique globo-series ganglioside isolated from human teratocarcinoma cells. EMBO J 1983; 2(12): 2355-61.
[PMID: 6141938]

[85]   Kannagi R, Levery SB, Hakomori S. Blood group H antigen with globo-series structure. Isolation and characterization from human blood group O erythrocytes. FEBS Lett 1984; 175(2): 397-401.
[http://dx.doi.org/10.1016/0014-5793(84)80776-0] [PMID: 6479351]

[86]   Bremer EG, Levery SB, Sonnino S, *et al.* Characterization of a glycosphingolipid antigen defined by the monoclonal antibody MBr1 expressed in normal and neoplastic epithelial cells of human mammary

gland. J Biol Chem 1984; 259(23): 14773-7.
[PMID: 6501317]

[87]   Clausen H, Watanabe K, Kannagi R, *et al.* Blood group A glycolipid (Ax) with globo-series structure
which is specific for blood group A$_1$ erythrocytes: one of the chemical bases for A$_1$ and A$_2$ distinction.
Biochem Biophys Res Commun 1984; 124(2): 523-9.
[http://dx.doi.org/10.1016/0006-291X(84)91585-7] [PMID: 6497890]

[88]   Levery SB, Salyan ME, Steele SJ, *et al.* A revised structure for the disialosyl globo-series gangliosides
of human erythrocytes and chicken skeletal muscle. Arch Biochem Biophys 1994; 312(1): 125-34.
[http://dx.doi.org/10.1006/abbi.1994.1290] [PMID: 8031119]

[89]   Sekine M, Taya C, Kikkawa Y, *et al.* Regulation of mouse kidney tubular epithelial cell-specific
expression of core 2 GlcNAc transferase. Eur J Biochem 2001; 268(4): 1129-35.
[http://dx.doi.org/10.1046/j.1432-1327.2001.01980.x] [PMID: 11179979]

[90]   Suzuki A, Yoshioka S, Sekine M, Yonekawa H, Takenaka M, Kannagi R. Core 2 GlcNAc transferase
and kidney tubular cell-specific expression. Glycoconj J 2004; 20(3): 151-6.
[http://dx.doi.org/10.1023/B:GLYC.0000024247.24605.97] [PMID: 15090728]

[91]   Schrump DS, Furukawa K, Yamaguchi H, Lloyd KO, Old LJ. Recognition of galactosylgloboside by
monoclonal antibodies derived from patients with primary lung cancer. Proc Natl Acad Sci USA 1988;
85(12): 4441-5.
[http://dx.doi.org/10.1073/pnas.85.12.4441] [PMID: 2837767]

[92]   Suzuki Y, Haraguchi N, Takahashi H, *et al.* SSEA-3 as a novel amplifying cancer cell surface marker
in colorectal cancers. Int J Oncol 2013; 42(1): 161-7.
[PMID: 23175153]

[93]   Gottschling S, Jensen K, Warth A, *et al.* Stage-specific embryonic antigen-4 is expressed in basaloid
lung cancer and associated with poor prognosis. Eur Respir J 2013; 41(3): 656-63.
[http://dx.doi.org/10.1183/09031936.00225711] [PMID: 22743677]

[94]   Lou YW, Wang PY, Yeh SC, *et al.* Stage-specific embryonic antigen-4 as a potential therapeutic target
in glioblastoma multiforme and other cancers. Proc Natl Acad Sci USA 2014; 111(7): 2482-7.
[http://dx.doi.org/10.1073/pnas.1400283111] [PMID: 24550271]

[95]   Chang WW, Lee CH, Lee P, *et al.* Expression of Globo H and SSEA3 in breast cancer stem cells and
the involvement of fucosyl transferases 1 and 2 in Globo H synthesis. Proc Natl Acad Sci USA 2008;
105(33): 11667-72.
[http://dx.doi.org/10.1073/pnas.0804979105] [PMID: 18685093]

[96]   Noto Z, Yoshida T, Okabe M, *et al.* CD44 and SSEA-4 positive cells in an oral cancer cell line HSC-4
possess cancer stem-like cell characteristics. Oral Oncol 2013; 49(8): 787-95.
[http://dx.doi.org/10.1016/j.oraloncology.2013.04.012] [PMID: 23768762]

[97]   Mao XG, Zhang X, Xue XY, *et al.* Brain tumor stem-like cells identified by neural stem cell marker
CD15. Transl Oncol 2009; 2(4): 247-57.
[http://dx.doi.org/10.1593/tlo.09136] [PMID: 19956386]

[98]   Son MJ, Woolard K, Nam DH, Lee J, Fine HA. SSEA-1 is an enrichment marker for tumor-initiating
cells in human glioblastoma. Cell Stem Cell 2009; 4(5): 440-52.

[http://dx.doi.org/10.1016/j.stem.2009.03.003] [PMID: 19427293]

[99]   Read TA, Fogarty MP, Markant SL, *et al.* Identification of CD15 as a marker for tumor-propagating cells in a mouse model of medulloblastoma. Cancer Cell 2009; 15(2): 135-47.
[http://dx.doi.org/10.1016/j.ccr.2008.12.016] [PMID: 19185848]

[100] Ward RJ, Lee L, Graham K, *et al.* Multipotent CD15+ cancer stem cells in patched-1-deficient mouse medulloblastoma. Cancer Res 2009; 69(11): 4682-90.
[http://dx.doi.org/10.1158/0008-5472.CAN-09-0342] [PMID: 19487286]

[101] Andrews PW, Goodfellow PN, Shevinsky LH, Bronson DL, Knowles BB. Cell-surface antigens of a clonal human embryonal carcinoma cell line: morphological and antigenic differentiation in culture. Int J Cancer 1982; 29(5): 523-31.
[http://dx.doi.org/10.1002/ijc.2910290507] [PMID: 7095898]

[102] Andrews PW, Banting G, Damjanov I, Arnaud D, Avner P. Three monoclonal antibodies defining distinct differentiation antigens associated with different high molecular weight polypeptides on the surface of human embryonal carcinoma cells. Hybridoma 1984; 3(4): 347-61.
[http://dx.doi.org/10.1089/hyb.1984.3.347] [PMID: 6396197]

[103] Badcock G, Pigott C, Goepel J, Andrews PW. The human embryonal carcinoma marker antigen TRA-1-60 is a sialylated keratan sulfate proteoglycan. Cancer Res 1999; 59(18): 4715-9.
[PMID: 10493530]

[104] Natunen S, Satomaa T, Pitkänen V, *et al.* The binding specificity of the marker antibodies Tra-1-60 and Tra-1-81 reveals a novel pluripotency-associated type 1 lactosamine epitope. Glycobiology 2011; 21(9): 1125-30.
[http://dx.doi.org/10.1093/glycob/cwq209] [PMID: 21159783]

[105] Rettig WJ, Cordon-Cardo C, Ng JS, Oettgen HF, Old LJ, Lloyd KO. High-molecular-weight glycoproteins of human teratocarcinoma defined by monoclonal antibodies to carbohydrate determinants. Cancer Res 1985; 45(2): 815-21.
[PMID: 2578310]

[106] Fukuda MN, Bothner B, Lloyd KO, Rettig WJ, Tiller PR, Dell A. Structures of glycosphingolipids isolated from human embryonal carcinoma cells. The presence of mono- and disialosyl glycolipids with blood group type 1 sequence. J Biol Chem 1986; 261(11): 5145-53.
[PMID: 3514610]

[107] Tang C, Lee AS, Volkmer JP, *et al.* An antibody against SSEA-5 glycan on human pluripotent stem cells enables removal of teratoma-forming cells. Nat Biotechnol 2011; 29(9): 829-34.
[http://dx.doi.org/10.1038/nbt.1947] [PMID: 21841799]

[108] Metzgar RS, Gaillard MT, Levine SJ, Tuck FL, Bossen EH, Borowitz MJ. Antigens of human pancreatic adenocarcinoma cells defined by murine monoclonal antibodies. Cancer Res 1982; 42(2): 601-8.
[PMID: 7034925]

[109] Craig EA, Austin AF, Vaillancourt RR, Barnett JV, Camenisch TD. TGFβ2-mediated production of hyaluronan is important for the induction of epicardial cell differentiation and invasion. Exp Cell Res 2010; 316(20): 3397-405.
[http://dx.doi.org/10.1016/j.yexcr.2010.07.006] [PMID: 20633555]

[110] Chow G, Tauler J, Mulshine JL. Cytokines and growth factors stimulate hyaluronan production: role of hyaluronan in epithelial to mesenchymal-like transition in non-small cell lung cancer. J Biomed Biotechnol 2010; 2010: 485468.

[111] Zhang H, Meng F, Wu S, *et al*. Engagement of I-branching β-1, 6-N-acetylglucosaminyltransferase 2 in breast cancer metastasis and TGF-β signaling. Cancer Res 2011; 71(14): 4846-56.
[http://dx.doi.org/10.1158/0008-5472.CAN-11-0414] [PMID: 21750175]

[112] Xu Q, Isaji T, Lu Y, *et al*. Roles of N-acetylglucosaminyltransferase III in epithelial-to-mesenchymal transition induced by transforming growth factor β1 (TGF-β1) in epithelial cell lines. J Biol Chem 2012; 287(20): 16563-74.
[http://dx.doi.org/10.1074/jbc.M111.262154] [PMID: 22451656]

[113] Pinho SS, Oliveira P, Cabral J, *et al*. Loss and recovery of Mgat3 and GnT-III Mediated E-cadherin N-glycosylation is a mechanism involved in epithelial-mesenchymal-epithelial transitions. PLoS One 2012; 7(3): e33191.
[http://dx.doi.org/10.1371/journal.pone.0033191] [PMID: 22427986]

[114] Kim J, Villadsen R, Sørlie T, *et al*. Tumor initiating but differentiated luminal-like breast cancer cells are highly invasive in the absence of basal-like activity. Proc Natl Acad Sci USA 2012; 109(16): 6124-9.
[http://dx.doi.org/10.1073/pnas.1203203109] [PMID: 22454501]

[115] Battula VL, Shi Y, Evans KW, *et al*. Ganglioside GD2 identifies breast cancer stem cells and promotes tumorigenesis. J Clin Invest 2012; 122(6): 2066-78.
[http://dx.doi.org/10.1172/JCI59735] [PMID: 22585577]

[116] Gupta V, Bhinge KN, Hosain SB, *et al*. Ceramide glycosylation by glucosylceramide synthase selectively maintains the properties of breast cancer stem cells. J Biol Chem 2012; 287(44): 37195-205.
[http://dx.doi.org/10.1074/jbc.M112.396390] [PMID: 22936806]

[117] Okuda H, Kobayashi A, Xia B, *et al*. Hyaluronan synthase HAS2 promotes tumor progression in bone by stimulating the interaction of breast cancer stem-like cells with macrophages and stromal cells. Cancer Res 2012; 72(2): 537-47.
[http://dx.doi.org/10.1158/0008-5472.CAN-11-1678] [PMID: 22113945]

[118] Li S, Mo C, Peng Q, *et al*. Cell surface glycan alterations in epithelial mesenchymal transition process of Huh7 hepatocellular carcinoma cell. PLoS One 2013; 8(8): e71273.
[http://dx.doi.org/10.1371/journal.pone.0071273] [PMID: 23977005]

[119] Swindall AF, Londoño-Joshi AI, Schultz MJ, Fineberg N, Buchsbaum DJ, Bellis SL. ST6Gal-I protein expression is upregulated in human epithelial tumors and correlates with stem cell markers in normal tissues and colon cancer cell lines. Cancer Res 2013; 73(7): 2368-78.
[http://dx.doi.org/10.1158/0008-5472.CAN-12-3424] [PMID: 23358684]

[120] Chen CY, Jan YH, Juan YH, *et al*. Fucosyltransferase 8 as a functional regulator of nonsmall cell lung cancer. Proc Natl Acad Sci USA 2013; 110(2): 630-5.
[http://dx.doi.org/10.1073/pnas.1220425110] [PMID: 23267084]

[121] Kim SJ, Chung TW, Choi HJ, *et al*. Ganglioside GM3 participates in the TGF-β1-induced epithelial-

mesenchymal transition of human lens epithelial cells. Biochem J 2013; 449(1): 241-51.
[http://dx.doi.org/10.1042/BJ20120189] [PMID: 23050851]

[122] Liang YJ, Ding Y, Levery SB, Lobaton M, Handa K, Hakomori SI. Differential expression profiles of glycosphingolipids in human breast cancer stem cells *vs.* cancer non-stem cells. Proc Natl Acad Sci USA 2013; 110(13): 4968-73.
[http://dx.doi.org/10.1073/pnas.1302825110] [PMID: 23479608]

[123] Guo J, Li X, Tan Z, Lu W, Yang G, Guan F. Alteration of N-glycans and expression of their related glycogenes in the epithelial-mesenchymal transition of HCV29 bladder epithelial cells. Molecules 2014; 19(12): 20073-90.
[http://dx.doi.org/10.3390/molecules191220073] [PMID: 25470275]

[124] Huang Q, Miller MR, Schappet J, Henry MD. The glycosyltransferase LARGE2 is repressed by Snail and ZEB1 in prostate cancer. Cancer Biol Ther 2015; 16(1): 125-36.
[http://dx.doi.org/10.4161/15384047.2014.987078] [PMID: 25455932]

[125] Li N, Xu H, Fan K, *et al.* Altered β1,6-GlcNAc branched N-glycans impair TGF-β-mediated epithelial-to-mesenchymal transition through Smad signalling pathway in human lung cancer. J Cell Mol Med 2014; 18(10): 1975-91.
[http://dx.doi.org/10.1111/jcmm.12331] [PMID: 24913443]

[126] Tan Z, Lu W, Li X, *et al.* Altered N-Glycan expression profile in epithelial-to-mesenchymal transition of NMuMG cells revealed by an integrated strategy using mass spectrometry and glycogene and lectin microarray analysis. J Proteome Res 2014; 13(6): 2783-95.
[http://dx.doi.org/10.1021/pr401185z] [PMID: 24724545]

[127] Silvestri I, Testa F, Zappasodi R, *et al.* NEU4 is involved in glioblastoma stem cell survival. Cell Death Dis 2014; 5: e13812014.
[http://dx.doi.org/10.1038/cddis.2014.349] [PMID: 25144716]

[128] Terao N, Takamatsu S, Minehira T, *et al.* Fucosylation is a common glycosylation type in pancreatic cancer stem cell-like phenotypes. World J Gastroenterol 2015; 21(13): 3876-87.
[http://dx.doi.org/10.3748/wjg.v21.i13.3876] [PMID: 25852272]

[129] Desiderio V, Papagerakis P, Tirino V, *et al.* Increased fucosylation has a pivotal role in invasive and metastatic properties of head and neck cancer stem cells. Oncotarget 2015; 6(1): 71-84.
[PMID: 25428916]

[130] Kurcon T, Liu Z, Paradkar AV, *et al.* miRNA proxy approach reveals hidden functions of glycosylation. Proc Natl Acad Sci USA 2015; 112(23): 7327-32.
[http://dx.doi.org/10.1073/pnas.1502076112] [PMID: 26015571]

Tumor Endothelial Cells and Cancer Progression

Kyoko Hida[1,*], Nako Maishi[1], Dorcas A. Annan[1] and Yasuhiro Hida[2]

[1] *Vascular Biology, Frontier Research Unit, Institute for Genetic Medicine, Hokkaido University, Sapporo, Japan*

[2] *Department of Cardiovascular and Thoracic Surgery, Hokkaido University Graduate School of Medicine, Sapporo, Japan*

Abstract: Tumor growth and metastasis are facilitated by the formation of new blood vessels, a process known as angiogenesis. The blood vessels formed around the tumor supply it with oxygen and nutrients, which together support its progression. Moreover, the newly formed blood vessels serve as channels through which tumor cells metastasize to distant organs. Tumor blood vessels, and especially the endothelial cells lining tumor blood vessels (tumor endothelial cells, TECs), have therefore gained interest as targets in cancer therapy. Although newly formed tumor blood vessels originate from pre-existing, normal vessels, they have a distinctively abnormal phenotype, including important morphological alterations. The balance between the angiogenic stimulators and inhibitors regulates angiogenesis in the tumor microenvironment. Furthermore, TECs constitute a heterogeneous population, exhibiting characteristics induced largely by tumor microenvironmental factors. In this chapter we review recent studies on TEC abnormalities regarding to cancer progression and consider the therapeutic implications thereof.

Keywords: Angiogenesis, Angiogenic factor, Anti-angiogenic therapy, Basement membrane, Blood vessel, Cancer, Drug resistance, Endothelial cell, Heterogeneity, Hypoxia, Invasion, Metastasis, Migration, Pericyte, Side effect, Tumor, Tumor angiogenesis, VEGF.

* **Corresponding author Kyoko Hida:** Vascular Biology, Frontier Research Unit, Institute for Genetic Medicine, Hokkaido University, N15, W7, Kita-ku, Sapporo, 060-0815, Japan; Tel: +81-11-706-4315; Fax: +81-11-706-4325; E-mail: khida@igm.hokudai.ac.jp.

TUMOR ANGIOGENESIS

Angiogenesis leads to the formation of new blood vessels and is essential for tumor progression. Tumor blood vessels supply the tumor with needed oxygen and nutrients, in addition to removing waste products from tumor tissue. However, tumor vessels also provide a route to metastasis [1, 2]. The endothelial cells that line tumor blood vessels (TECs) have emerged as important targets of angiogenic inhibitors (anti-angiogenic therapy) and provide a strategy for cancer treatment, with many anti-angiogenic drugs developed and tested to date [3]. The basis for pursuing this therapy can be summarized as follows: i) The survival of a large population of tumor cells depends on a few TECs, such that targeting TECs may be more efficient than targeting tumor cells. ii) Since TECs exhibit similar characteristics regardless of their tumor of origin, a single, effective anti-angiogenic drug could be used to treat many forms of cancer. iii) It was thought that TECs are genetically stable unlike tumor cells, and therefore do not become drug resistant. However, recent studies have shown that TECs from primary tumor sites differ from normal endothelial cells (NECs) and their makeup in various tumor types is heterogeneous. Moreover, while anti-angiogenic drugs were thought to be less toxic than other cytotoxic drugs, it is now clear that they may induce severe side effects, such as lethal hemoptysis [4, 5] and intestinal perforation [6, 7]. Accordingly, an important goal in cancer therapy is to develop novel and safer tumor anti-angiogenic agents, which in turn depends on a thorough understanding of the biology of TECs.

TUMOR BLOOD VESSELS ARE MORPHOLOGICALLY ABNORMAL

Tumor blood vessels differ in many ways from normal blood vessels (Fig. **1a**). Specifically, tumor vessels are not organized in the same hierarchal branching pattern (*i.e.*, from arteries to capillaries and then veins) as the normal vasculature [8]. Their underlying basement membranes are of varying thicknesses, and their TECs do not form regular monolayers [9], unlike in normal blood vessels [10]. Although pericytes are present, they form abnormally loose association with TECs [11]. Consequently, tumor blood vessels are leaky. Other abnormalities of tumor blood vessels have been attributed to the unbalanced expression of angiogenic factors and inhibitors (Fig. **1b**). In addition to the above characteristics, tumor blood vessels are often immature morphologically, The high interstitial fluid pressure in cancer causes vessel collapse and blood flow is compromised. Furthermore, tumor vessels show chaotic blood flow and they are leaky because of the loose interconnections in endothelium [12]. These features of tumor vasculature may be one of reason why cancers are usually hypoxia even though they are highly vascularized. Hypoxia in cancer is the cause of resistance to radiation therapy [13].

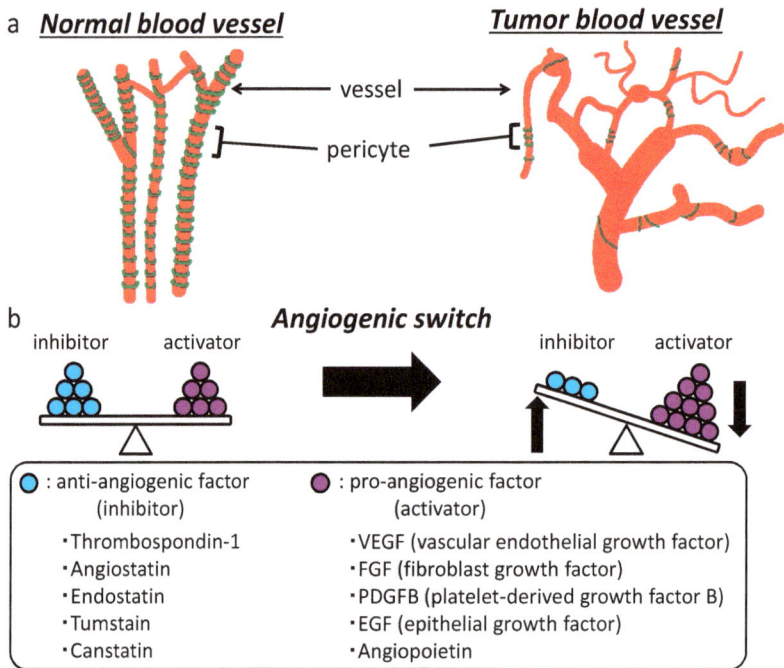

Fig. (1). Differences in the blood vessels of tumors and normal tissue.
(a) Tumor vessels show excessive branching but lack the arteriole-capillary-venule hierarchy. As a result, blood flow through these vessels is chaotic. Resident pericytes in tumors associate with endothelial cells loosely. **(b)** Tumors are characterized by imbalances between the levels of pro-angiogenic (activators) and anti-angiogenic (inhibitors) factors. The up-regulation of activators *vs.* inhibitors causes an angiogenic switch in the tumors.

TECs are morphologically irregular, with long cytoplasmic projections extending across the lumen, whereas NEC are uniform. The endothelial gaps and transcellular fenestrae in the walls of tumor blood vessels result in hemorrhage and plasma leakage, two common properties of tumors. Moreover, they allow filling in by adjacent tumor cells and provide a mechanism for tumor cell intravasation, an initial step in metastasis [14].

DIFFERENCES BETWEEN TUMOR ENDOTHELIAL CELLS AND NORMAL ENDOTHELIAL CELLS

Phenotypic differences at the molecular and functional levels have been identified in TECs and NECs isolated from tumor and normal tissue, respectively. However, until recently, few studies had examined the features of isolated TECs. Instead, for many years most studies on tumor angiogenesis has been done by using NECs, such as human umbilical vein endothelial cells. TECs can be isolated by immunomagnetic sorting using an antibody against endothelial cell markers such as CD31, ICAM-2, but possible contamination by tumor cells and fibroblasts has been considered to be a bottleneck for TEC culture. Contamination of human tumor cells can be eliminated using diphtheria toxin (DT) from mouse TEC, isolated from a human tumor xenografted into mice [15]. The use of DT was based on the fact that heparin-binding epidermal growth factor (HB-EGF) is a receptor of DT in human but not mouse cells, and DT is toxic for human cells expressing HB-EGF but not mouse cells [16]. Nonetheless, obtaining enough TECs to allow their study remains difficult because these cells constitute only a small cell fraction within tumor tissues.

Recent studies have demonstrated molecular differences between TECs and NECs [17, 18]. For example, our lab has shown that isolated TECs exhibit several abnormalities compared with NECs [15, 19], including differences in their responsiveness to growth factors such as EGF [20], adrenomedullin [21], and vascular endothelial growth factor (VEGF) [22], all of which contribute to the pro-angiogenic phenotype of TECs. VEGF stimulates the migration of TECs and enhances their survival in an autocrine manner. This VEGF autocrine loop also contributes to the resistance of TECs to serum starvation, which is absent in NECs [22]. In addition, several cytogenetic abnormalities, such as aneuploidy and abnormal centrosomes, have been detected in TECs from mouse tumors [15] and human renal carcinomas [23]. These abnormalities were confirmed to be not due to tumor cell contaminants. Aneuploidy is an indicator of genetic instability and likely explains the frequently observed resistance of TECs to chemotherapeutic agents [24, 25], including the vincristine resistance of TECs from a renal carcinoma [24], the 5-fluorouracil and adriamycin resistance of TECs from a hepatocellular carcinoma [25, 26], and the tumor-derived VEGF mediated resistance of TECs to paclitaxel [26]. However, the actual mechanism underlying the drug resistance of TECs remains unknown.

HETEROGENEITY OF NORMAL ENDOTHELIAL CELLS

Endothelial cell heterogeneity may be morphological, functional, or related to gene expression. For example, the rolling velocity and arrest frequency of leukocytes at NEC junctions is different than at central areas [27]. Inter-organ differences in NECs have also been reported [28]. In pre-existing blood vessels, stem-like endothelial cells with a pro-angiogenic phenotype have been identified [29]. Additionally, in rat brain blood vessels, particularly at the single-cell level, P-gp and endothelial barrier antigen are heterogeneously expressed, suggesting a lack of uniformity in the blood-brain barrier [30].

TEC HETEROGENEITY

Many examples of TEC heterogeneity exist [15, 17, 24, 31]. Within the tumor vasculature, the morphology and pericyte coverage of tumor blood vessels vary depending on tumor type and progression stage [28, 32, 33]. Furthermore, these recently appreciated heterogeneities [34] differ between highly metastatic (HM) and low metastatic (LM) tumors. The blood vessels of HM tumors are more immature, with fewer pericytes, than the blood vessels of LM tumors [34]. These features contribute to the higher hypoxic nature of HM than LM tumors. TECs isolated from HM tumors (HM-TECs) have a higher proliferative index, motility, and sensitivity to VEGF, more abundant extracellular matrix (ECM), and greater invasive ability than their LM counterparts (LM-TECs). In addition, in HM-TECs several angiogenesis-related genes, such as VEGFR-1, VEGFR-2, VEGF, and the genes encoding the PI3K/Akt signaling pathway, which is crucial in angiogenesis, are up-regulated [35, 36].

Features that contribute to the higher invasive potential of HM-TECs and distinguish them from LM-TECs include the higher level of Akt phosphorylation under basal conditions and the up-regulation of gelatinase/collagenase IV matrix metalloproteases (MMP-2 and MMP-9) subsequent to PI3K/Akt pathway activation. During tumor neovascularization, MMPs are used by TECs to breach the basement membrane and degrade the ECM, thus allowing TEC migration to the tumor. All of these events promote tumor metastasis.

DRUG RESISTANCE AND CYTOGENETIC ABNORMALITIES IN HM-TECS

As noted above, TECs are resistant to several anti-cancer drugs. Tumors in which the expression of MDR1/P-gp is up-regulated are resistant to paclitaxel [26]. Higher levels of MDR1 mRNA are detected in HM-TECs than in LM-TECs. Complex abnormal karyotypes and high aneuploidy rates are associated with cancer cells containing multidrug resistance genes [37]. Our group has reported that, under the same culture conditions, TECs are karyotypically aneuploid, whereas NECs are diploid [15, 23, 38]. In addition, a GTG-banding study demonstrated that HM-TECs have more complex abnormal karyotypes than LM-TECs [34]. These cytogenetic abnormalities may contribute to HM-TEC drug resistance. The differences between HM-TECs and LM-TECs are summarized in Table **1**.

Table 1. Differences between HM-TECs and LM-TECs.

	The characteristics of TECs in highly metastatic compared to low metastatic tumors
Angiogenesis-related genes	Up-regulation of vascular endothelial growth factor (VEGF)-A, VEGF-receptor R1 and R2, hypoxia-inducible factor-1α, CXCL12
Pro-anigogenic phenotype	Higher proliferation rate Faster motility
Invasion-related genes	Up-regulation of matrix metalloproteases (MMP)-2, MMP-9 Down-regulation of tissue inhibitor of metalloproteinase-1
Drug resistance	Up-regulation of multi drug resistance gene (MDR-1) Resistance to anti-cancer drugs (5-fluorouracil, paclitaxel)
Stemness	Up-regulation of Sca-1, CD90, and CD133 Enhanced sphere forming activity Increased bone differentiation activity
Chromosomal abnormalities	Higher aneuploidy rates Karyotypic abnormalities

MECHANISMS OF TEC HETEROGENEITY

Interactions between tumor cells and stromal cells facilitate tumor progression, tumor malignancy, and metastasis. Indeed, in NECs co-cultured with HM tumor cells, pro-angiogenic genes are up-regulated and phenotypic changes typical of TECs are observed [34], suggesting that tumor-secreted factors adversely influence their associated stromal cells.

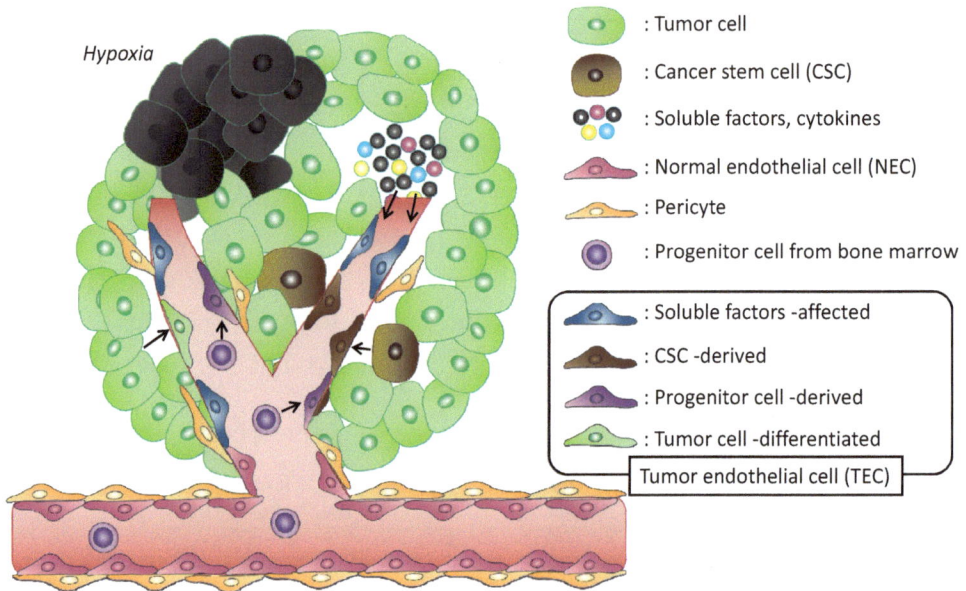

Fig. (2). Mechanism of TEC heterogeneity. TECs are exposed to the factors-secreted from tumor cells or stromal cells. Cancer stem cells, tumor cells, and vascular progenitor cells from bone marrow may be involved in neo-vessel formation.

Hypoxia may also contribute to the pro-angiogenic phenotype of HM-TECs. A rapidly growing tumor cells will soon deplete nutrients and oxygen, resulting in hypoxia and necrosis. And, the immature, abnormal, and leaky, tumor blood vessels may be easily compressed by the high tissue pressure within the tumor, which also leads to hypoxia [39, 40]. In HM tumors, hypoxia induces excessive VEGF production, vascular permeability, and it may cause genetic instability in HM-TECs [41]. The increased vascular permeability compromises blood flow in the blood vessels of HM tumors, which further decreases nutrient and oxygen delivery, thus causing the physiological stress of the tumor. The persisting hypoxia together with the secretion of cytokines such as VEGF and CXCL12, promotes tumor revascularization, by inducing the mobilization of bone marrow derived endothelial progenitor cells to cancer [42] (Fig. **2**). The heterogeneity of TECs has also been accounted for the origin of these cells. Among the cells thought to be capable of differentiating into TECs are glioblastoma cells [43, 44], although a recent study showed that glioblastoma cells give rise to pericytes, not endothelial cells [45]. The transdifferentiation of lymphoma cells into TECs was also proposed to underlie TEC heterogeneity [46]. However, these findings are not supported by our observations in studies of a cross-species model (human tumor and mouse endothelial cells). The full range of mechanisms that account for TEC heterogeneity remain to be determined in further studies.

CONCLUSION

TECs differ from NECs morphologically, behaviorally, and in their gene profile patterns. Contrary to previous assumptions, TECs are not genetically stable and are therefore likely to develop resistance to chemotherapeutic agents. Indeed, it is now evident that cytogenetic abnormalities are one of the main feature of the TECs of non-hematopoietic solid tumors. This discovery has important implications, given that, as in chemotherapeutic resistance of the tumor, resistance to anti-angiogenic therapies will result in treatment failure. However, stromal cells in the tumor microenvironment may also be abnormal, and they can be an additional target for cancer therapy. Further studies on abnormalities of TECs and the various cell types that make up cancer are required to develop novel anti-angiogenic therapies.

FUNDING

This work was supported by Grants-in-Aid for Scientific Research from the Ministry of Education, Science, and Culture of Japan (to K. Hida, Y. Hida, and N. Maishi) and by grants from the Akiyama Foundation (to K. Hida).

DISCLOSURE

Part of this chapter has been previously published in International Journal of Clinical Oncology. April 2016, Volume 21, Issue 2, pp 206-212. DOI

10.1007/s10147-016-0957-1.

CONFLICT OF INTEREST

The authors confirm that they have no conflict of interest to declare for this publication.

ACKNOWLEDGEMENTS

We thank the members of the Department of Vascular Biology, Institute for Genetic Medicine, Hokkaido University, and Dr. Shindoh for helpful discussions.

REFERENCES

[1]   Folkman J. Tumor angiogenesis: therapeutic implications. N Engl J Med 1971; 285(21): 1182-6.
[http://dx.doi.org/10.1056/NEJM197111182852108] [PMID: 4938153]

[2]   Folkman J, Kerbel R. Role of angiogenesis in tumor growth and metastasis. Semin Oncol 2002; 29(6) (Suppl. 16): 15-8.
[http://dx.doi.org/10.1016/S0093-7754(02)70065-1] [PMID: 12516034]

[3]   Folkman J. Angiogenesis: an organizing principle for drug discovery? Nat Rev Drug Discov 2007; 6(4): 273-86.
[http://dx.doi.org/10.1038/nrd2115] [PMID: 17396134]

[4]   Johnson DH, Fehrenbacher L, Novotny WF, *et al.* Randomized phase II trial comparing bevacizumab plus carboplatin and paclitaxel with carboplatin and paclitaxel alone in previously untreated locally advanced or metastatic non-small-cell lung cancer. J Clin Oncol 2004; 22(11): 2184-91.
[http://dx.doi.org/10.1200/JCO.2004.11.022] [PMID: 15169807]

[5]   Keedy VL, Sandler AB. Inhibition of angiogenesis in the treatment of non-small cell lung cancer. Cancer Sci 2007; 98(12): 1825-30.
[http://dx.doi.org/10.1111/j.1349-7006.2007.00620.x] [PMID: 17892508]

[6]   Kindler HL, Friberg G, Singh DA, *et al.* Phase II trial of bevacizumab plus gemcitabine in patients with advanced pancreatic cancer. J Clin Oncol 2005; 23(31): 8033-40.
[http://dx.doi.org/10.1200/JCO.2005.01.9661] [PMID: 16258101]

[7]   Saif MW, Elfiky A, Salem RR. Gastrointestinal perforation due to bevacizumab in colorectal cancer. Ann Surg Oncol 2007; 14(6): 1860-9.
[http://dx.doi.org/10.1245/s10434-006-9337-9] [PMID: 17356952]

[8]   McDonald DM, Choyke PL. Imaging of angiogenesis: from microscope to clinic. Nat Med 2003; 9(6): 713-25.
[http://dx.doi.org/10.1038/nm0603-713] [PMID: 12778170]

[9]   Hashizume H, Baluk P, Morikawa S, *et al.* Openings between defective endothelial cells explain tumor vessel leakiness. Am J Pathol 2000; 156(4): 1363-80.
[http://dx.doi.org/10.1016/S0002-9440(10)65006-7] [PMID: 10751361]

[10] Kalluri R. Basement membranes: structure, assembly and role in tumour angiogenesis. Nat Rev Cancer 2003; 3(6): 422-33.
[http://dx.doi.org/10.1038/nrc1094] [PMID: 12778132]

[11] Baluk P, Hashizume H, McDonald DM. Cellular abnormalities of blood vessels as targets in cancer. Curr Opin Genet Dev 2005; 15(1): 102-11.
[http://dx.doi.org/10.1016/j.gde.2004.12.005] [PMID: 15661540]

[12] McDonald DM, Baluk P. Significance of blood vessel leakiness in cancer. Cancer Res 2002; 62(18): 5381-5.
[PMID: 12235011]

[13] Jain RK. Normalization of tumor vasculature: an emerging concept in antiangiogenic therapy. Science 2005; 307(5706): 58-62.
[http://dx.doi.org/10.1126/science.1104819] [PMID: 15637262]

[14] Chang YS, di Tomaso E, McDonald DM, Jones R, Jain RK, Munn LL. Mosaic blood vessels in tumors: frequency of cancer cells in contact with flowing blood. Proc Natl Acad Sci USA 2000; 97(26): 14608-13.
[http://dx.doi.org/10.1073/pnas.97.26.14608] [PMID: 11121063]

[15] Hida K, Hida Y, Amin DN, *et al.* Tumor-associated endothelial cells with cytogenetic abnormalities. Cancer Res 2004; 64(22): 8249-55.
[http://dx.doi.org/10.1158/0008-5472.CAN-04-1567] [PMID: 15548691]

[16] Arbiser JL, Raab G, Rohan RM, *et al.* Isolation of mouse stromal cells associated with a human tumor using differential diphtheria toxin sensitivity. Am J Pathol 1999; 155(3): 723-9.
[http://dx.doi.org/10.1016/S0002-9440(10)65171-1] [PMID: 10487830]

[17] St Croix B, Rago C, Velculescu V, *et al.* Genes expressed in human tumor endothelium. Science 2000; 289(5482): 1197-202.
[http://dx.doi.org/10.1126/science.289.5482.1197] [PMID: 10947988]

[18] Seaman S, Stevens J, Yang MY, Logsdon D, Graff-Cherry C, St Croix B. Genes that distinguish physiological and pathological angiogenesis. Cancer Cell 2007; 11(6): 539-54.
[http://dx.doi.org/10.1016/j.ccr.2007.04.017] [PMID: 17560335]

[19] Hida K, Klagsbrun M. A new perspective on tumor endothelial cells: unexpected chromosome and centrosome abnormalities. Cancer Res 2005; 65(7): 2507-10.
[http://dx.doi.org/10.1158/0008-5472.CAN-05-0002] [PMID: 15805239]

[20] Amin DN, Hida K, Bielenberg DR, Klagsbrun M. Tumor endothelial cells express epidermal growth factor receptor (EGFR) but not ErbB3 and are responsive to EGF and to EGFR kinase inhibitors. Cancer Res 2006; 66(4): 2173-80.
[http://dx.doi.org/10.1158/0008-5472.CAN-05-3387] [PMID: 16489018]

[21] Tsuchiya K, Hida K, Hida Y, *et al.* Adrenomedullin antagonist suppresses tumor formation in renal cell carcinoma through inhibitory effects on tumor endothelial cells and endothelial progenitor mobilization. Int J Oncol 2010; 36(6): 1379-86.
[PMID: 20428760]

[22] Matsuda K, Ohga N, Hida Y, *et al.* Isolated tumor endothelial cells maintain specific character during

long-term culture. Biochem Biophys Res Commun 2010; 394(4): 947-54.
[http://dx.doi.org/10.1016/j.bbrc.2010.03.089] [PMID: 20302845]

[23]   Akino T, Hida K, Hida Y, *et al.* Cytogenetic abnormalities of tumor-associated endothelial cells in human malignant tumors. Am J Pathol 2009; 175(6): 2657-67.
[http://dx.doi.org/10.2353/ajpath.2009.090202] [PMID: 19875502]

[24]   Bussolati B, Deambrosis I, Russo S, Deregibus MC, Camussi G. Altered angiogenesis and survival in human tumor-derived endothelial cells. FASEB J 2003; 17(9): 1159-61.
[PMID: 12709414]

[25]   Xiong YQ, Sun HC, Zhang W, *et al.* Human hepatocellular carcinoma tumor-derived endothelial cells manifest increased angiogenesis capability and drug resistance compared with normal endothelial cells. Clin Cancer Res 2009; 15(15): 4838-46.
[http://dx.doi.org/10.1158/1078-0432.CCR-08-2780] [PMID: 19638466]

[26]   Akiyama K, Ohga N, Hida Y, *et al.* Tumor endothelial cells acquire drug resistance by MDR1 up-regulation *via* VEGF signaling in tumor microenvironment. Am J Pathol 2012; 180(3): 1283-93.
[http://dx.doi.org/10.1016/j.ajpath.2011.11.029] [PMID: 22245726]

[27]   Mundhekar AN, Bullard DC, Kucik DF. Intracellular heterogeneity in adhesiveness of endothelium affects early steps in leukocyte adhesion. Am J Physiol Cell Physiol 2006; 291(1): C130-7.
[http://dx.doi.org/10.1152/ajpcell.00261.2005] [PMID: 16769816]

[28]   Molema G. Heterogeneity in endothelial responsiveness to cytokines, molecular causes, and pharmacological consequences. Semin Thromb Hemost 2010; 36(3): 246-64.
[http://dx.doi.org/10.1055/s-0030-1253448] [PMID: 20490977]

[29]   Naito H, Kidoya H, Sakimoto S, Wakabayashi T, Takakura N. Identification and characterization of a resident vascular stem/progenitor cell population in preexisting blood vessels. EMBO J 2012; 31(4): 842-55.
[http://dx.doi.org/10.1038/emboj.2011.465] [PMID: 22179698]

[30]   Saubaméa B, Cochois-Guégan V, Cisternino S, Scherrmann JM. Heterogeneity in the rat brain vasculature revealed by quantitative confocal analysis of endothelial barrier antigen and P-glycoprotein expression. J Cereb Blood Flow Metab 2012; 32(1): 81-92.
[http://dx.doi.org/10.1038/jcbfm.2011.109] [PMID: 21792241]

[31]   Dudley AC, Khan ZA, Shih SC, *et al.* Calcification of multipotent prostate tumor endothelium. Cancer Cell 2008; 14(3): 201-11.
[http://dx.doi.org/10.1016/j.ccr.2008.06.017] [PMID: 18772110]

[32]   Langenkamp E, Molema G. Microvascular endothelial cell heterogeneity: general concepts and pharmacological consequences for anti-angiogenic therapy of cancer. Cell Tissue Res 2009; 335(1): 205-22.
[http://dx.doi.org/10.1007/s00441-008-0642-4] [PMID: 18677515]

[33]   Nagy JA, Dvorak HF. Heterogeneity of the tumor vasculature: the need for new tumor blood vessel type-specific targets. Clin Exp Metastasis 2012; 29(7): 657-62.
[http://dx.doi.org/10.1007/s10585-012-9500-6] [PMID: 22692562]

[34]   Ohga N, Ishikawa S, Maishi N, *et al.* Heterogeneity of tumor endothelial cells: comparison between

tumor endothelial cells isolated from high- and low-metastatic tumors. Am J Pathol 2012; 180(3): 1294-307.
[http://dx.doi.org/10.1016/j.ajpath.2011.11.035] [PMID: 22245217]

[35] Bussolati B, Assenzio B, Deregibus MC, Camussi G. The proangiogenic phenotype of human tumor-derived endothelial cells depends on thrombospondin-1 downregulation *via* phosphatidylinositol 3-kinase/Akt pathway. J Mol Med 2006; 84(10): 852-63.
[http://dx.doi.org/10.1007/s00109-006-0075-z] [PMID: 16924472]

[36] Adya R, Tan BK, Punn A, Chen J, Randeva HS. Visfatin induces human endothelial VEGF and MMP-2/9 production *via* MAPK and PI3K/Akt signalling pathways: novel insights into visfatin-induced angiogenesis. Cardiovasc Res 2008; 78(2): 356-65.
[http://dx.doi.org/10.1093/cvr/cvm111] [PMID: 18093986]

[37] Duensing S, Münger K. Human papillomaviruses and centrosome duplication errors: modeling the origins of genomic instability. Oncogene 2002; 21(40): 6241-8.
[http://dx.doi.org/10.1038/sj.onc.1205709] [PMID: 12214255]

[38] Hida K, Hida Y, Shindoh M. Understanding tumor endothelial cell abnormalities to develop ideal anti-angiogenic therapies. Cancer Sci 2008; 99(3): 459-66.
[http://dx.doi.org/10.1111/j.1349-7006.2007.00704.x] [PMID: 18167133]

[39] Sato Y. Persistent vascular normalization as an alternative goal of anti-angiogenic cancer therapy. Cancer Sci 2011; 102(7): 1253-6.
[http://dx.doi.org/10.1111/j.1349-7006.2011.01929.x] [PMID: 21401807]

[40] Helfrich I, Scheffrahn I, Bartling S, *et al.* Resistance to antiangiogenic therapy is directed by vascular phenotype, vessel stabilization, and maturation in malignant melanoma. J Exp Med 2010; 207(3): 491-503.
[http://dx.doi.org/10.1084/jem.20091846] [PMID: 20194633]

[41] Taylor SM, Nevis KR, Park HL, *et al.* Angiogenic factor signaling regulates centrosome duplication in endothelial cells of developing blood vessels. Blood 2010; 116(16): 3108-17.
[http://dx.doi.org/10.1182/blood-2010-01-266197] [PMID: 20664058]

[42] Gao D, Nolan D, McDonnell K, *et al.* Bone marrow-derived endothelial progenitor cells contribute to the angiogenic switch in tumor growth and metastatic progression. Biochim Biophys Acta 2009; 1796(1): 33-40.
[PMID: 19460418]

[43] Ricci-Vitiani L, Pallini R, Biffoni M, *et al.* Tumour vascularization *via* endothelial differentiation of glioblastoma stem-like cells. Nature 2010; 468(7325): 824-8.
[http://dx.doi.org/10.1038/nature09557] [PMID: 21102434]

[44] Wang R, Chadalavada K, Wilshire J, *et al.* Glioblastoma stem-like cells give rise to tumour endothelium. Nature 2010; 468(7325): 829-33.
[http://dx.doi.org/10.1038/nature09624] [PMID: 21102433]

[45] Cheng L, Huang Z, Zhou W, *et al.* Glioblastoma stem cells generate vascular pericytes to support vessel function and tumor growth. Cell 2013; 153(1): 139-52.
[http://dx.doi.org/10.1016/j.cell.2013.02.021] [PMID: 23540695]

[46]   Streubel B, Chott A, Huber D, *et al.* Lymphoma-specific genetic aberrations in microvascular endothelial cells in B-cell lymphomas. N Engl J Med 2004; 351(3): 250-9.
[http://dx.doi.org/10.1056/NEJMoa033153] [PMID: 15254283]

CHAPTER 4

Metastatic Cancer Stem Cell Niche and the Toll-like Receptor 4 (TLR4)-mediated Premetastatic Microenvironment

Takeshi Tomita[*], **Atsuko Deguchi**[*] and **Yoshiro Maru**

Department of Pharmacology, Tokyo Women's Medical University, Tokyo, Japan

Abstract: Cancer metastasis is one of the most crucial problems in the field of medical research. There are two types of approaches to find a new way to treat cancer metastasis; Targeting cancer stem cells, or stromal cells in the premetastatic phase. Interactions between these two elements synergistically enhance the survival of metastatic cancer cells and promote their re-growth in the distant organ. In this review, first we summarize the recent trends in cancer stem cell studies. Then, we discuss the premetastatic phase, based on our investigations. We also review various types of tumor-associated stromal cells (monocyte/macrophage, fibroblast, adipocyte, dendritic cell, neutrophil, and natural killer cell) in relations with the tumor microenvironment formation. Moreover, dormant tumor cells and circulating tumor cells are included in this review.

Keywords: Biglycan, CCL2, CCR2, Circulating tumor cell, Dormant cell, EMT, Eph, Ephrin A1, HMGB1, Inflammation, MD-2, Metalloprotease, Organ tropism, Premetastatic microenvironment, S100A8, SAA3, TGF-β, TLR4, TNFα, VEGF.

I. OVERVIEW

I-a. Outline of Tumor Metastasis

It is often said that tumor metastasis do not just happen. Actually, it is a sequence

---

[*] **Corresponding authors Takeshi Tomita and Atsuko Deguchi:** Department of Pharmacology, Tokyo Women's Medical University, 8-1 Kawada, Shinjuku, Tokyo, 162-8666, Japan; Tel/Fax: +81-3-5269-7417; Emails: tomitat@research.twmu.ac.jp, deguchi@research.twmu.ac.jp

Takanori Kawaguchi (Ed.)

of events including dissemination of tumor cells from (a) primary tumor formation, (b) local invasion, (c) intravasation, (d) cell survival during circulation in blood vessels, (e) extravasation, (f) settlement of tumor cells at distant organ, and (g) metastatic tumor regrowth. Every single step has been intensively scrutinized so that myriads of reports are available. The outline of "the premetastatic phase"/metastasis is shown in Fig. (**1**).

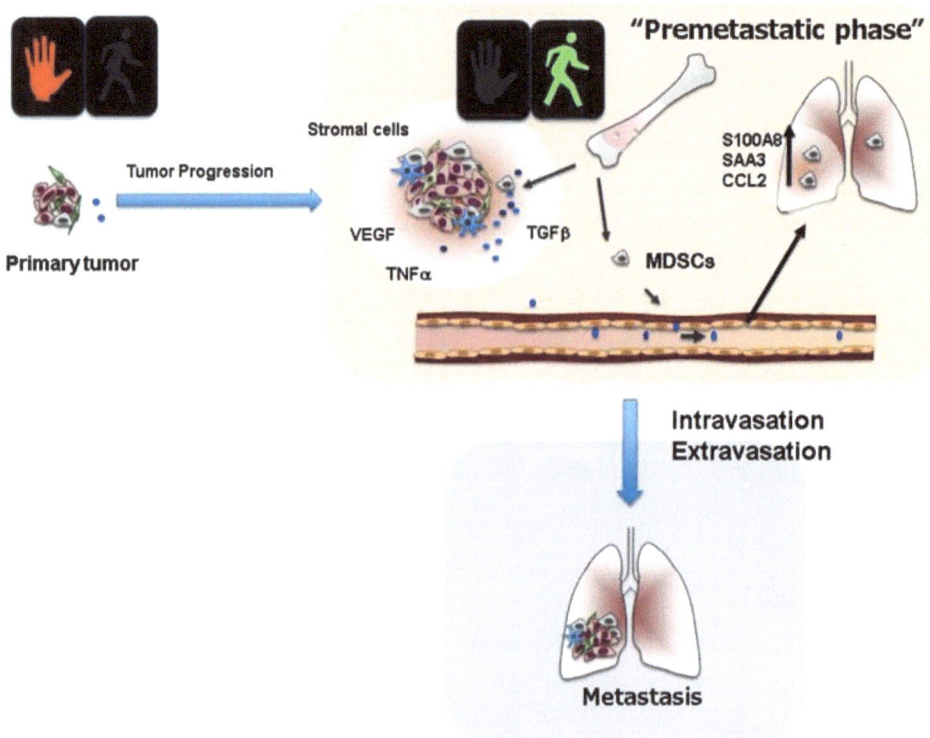

Fig. (1). Outline of the pre-metastatic phase.
The recruitment of myeloid-derived cells is a crucial step in metastasis. In the early phase of the primary tumor, it is not ready for myeloid-derived cells (monocytes, MDSCs) to recruit primary tumor sites and distant organs (in this case, lung; Don't walk). Once tumors develop certain size, the primary tumor microenvironment secretes cytokines/chemokines (*i.e.* VEGF, TNFα, and TGF-β) to supply to myeloid-derived cells. These cytokines can send a signal to myeloid-derived cells in bone marrow as "Walk".

Interestingly, different molecule comes forward with every single step toward metastasis. The data that knockdown of individual molecular, any given molecule highlighted in the research, by using knockout mouse or shRNA techniques seriously did hurt macroscopic metastasis indicate that tumor metastasis is a balance as subtle as on the edge of a cliff. In other words, since many molecules should be orchestrated for cancer metastasis, just disordered one piece is enough to make it incomplete.

For instance, cathepsins were indispensable to local tumor invasion [1, 2]. These metalloproteases were generated by macrophages upon stimulation of IL-4, secreted by tumor cells or T cells nearby [1, 3]. During intravasation, key molecules between tumor cells and macrophages became epidermal growth factor (EGF) and colony stimulating factor-1 (CSF-1) instcad [4]. Selectins prolonged the lifetime of tumor cells in the blood vessels [5]. Metadherin [6] and angiopoietin-like 4 (Angptl4 [7],) were necessary for tumor cells to extravasate in a distant organ. In order to commence the colonization, immigrated tumor cells required matrix metalloproteinase-9 (MMP-9) and stromal cell derived factor-1 (SDF-1) released from stromal cells [8]. Osteopontin from bone marrow derived cells were needed for further growth [9]. Vascular cell adhesion molecule-1 (VCAM-1) is one of the most hopeful therapeutic target molecules. VCAM-1 expressed on the metastatic tumor cells bound integrin $\alpha4\beta1$ on tumor-associated macrophages. With the ligand binding, the PI3K-Akt signaling pathway was activated, which caused dissemination of tumor cells in lungs [10, 11]. Again, these proteins are just a small portion. Different types of tumor cells may ask different kinds of molecular sets to metastasize, implying that custom-made regimens should be designed to prevent metastasis. Thus, this fact makes tumor treatment more painstaking.

Recent studies continue to shed light on potential therapeutic target molecules. Retinoic acid receptor responder protein 3 (RARRES3) was found out to be a metastasis suppressor. Phospholipase A1/A2 activity of this protein played an important role to keep tumor cells from initiating metastasis in the lungs [12]. Repression of thrombospondin-1, anti-angiogenic factor, was essential for tumor growth. Interestingly, an investigation uncovered that regulation of thrombospondin-1 in fibroblast was distinct from that in epithelial cells [13]. Cathepsin S promoted brain metastasis by cleaving junctional adhesion molecule-B (JAM-B) to facilitate tumor cells passing through the blood brain barrier [14]. A cathepsin S specific inhibitor, VBY-999, drastically reduced the chances of brain metastasis in the mouse model system. Nevertheless, the compound was ineffective to abrogate bone metastasis because cathepsin S was not involved in the process. Filopodium-like protrusions (FLP), defined as a cell morphological change observed in that matrigel-on-top culture, accounted for aggressiveness of tumor cells. FLP formation correlated with the cell proliferation rate in matrigel-on-top culture, but not monolayer culture, indicating that FLP structure was a prerequisite for tumor metastasis. It has been also shown that a carcinoma cell line with higher FLP frequency was more metastatic than lower FLP cell lines as evaluated by the tail vein injection assay. Intriguingly, two proteins, Rif and mDia2, which were necessary to form filopodia in monolayer culture, were shown to be required for FLP formation also, but not affect extravasation into the lung parenchyma in the mouse model study. The Rif and mDia2 ablated cell line exhibited an increase of micrometastasis, whereas the number of macro-metastasis was decreased [15]. Subsequent studies showed that integrin-linked kinase (ILK)/β-parvin/cofilin signaling axis governed FLP formation, and molecular function of Rif and mDia2 was determined to be the induction of actin monomer nucleation in the process. In addition, FLP formation preferentially occurred in cancer stem cells as judged by surface molecular marker expression pattern [16].

I-b. Traffic Accident Theory

If the tumor cell traffics in the blood flow are under control, the chances of metastasis should decrease drastically. Additionally, tumor cells are more vulnerable to therapeutic pressures (reagent, immune cells) in the blood flow than in the solid tissue because tumor cells are not guarded by the tumor-friendly cells or barriers. Many medical devices with cutting-edge technologies can capture circulating tumor cells in the blood flow. Therefore, we think that the dual approach (- devices and medicines) targeting circulating tumor cells will be one of the best options in the near future.

It is not uncommon to observe the fact that many tumor cells shed from the primary tumor are circulating in patients, but probably a tiny fraction of them stay alive on the metastatic site. According to an experimental system utilizing a mouse model, less than 3% of tail vein injected tumor cell regained micrometastasis and less than 0.02% finally attained macroscopic metastatic colonization. Here, to make matters simple, we wish to tumor metastasis liken to traffic accidents. We believe that this analogy is the best way we know to explain what is all about tumor metastasis for non-experts. In some cases, a particular crossroads are referred to be 'Deadly intersection', citing a couple of eye witnessed episodes of traffic accidents. Of course, this does not necessarily mean that all vehicles passing by are involved in the unfortunate events. Presumably, more than 99.9% of heavy traffic managed to leave without anything. In the real traffic accidents, people who were at a wrong time became a victim. Similarly, a tumor cell came across at a wrong time caused a tragedy. Just one accident in an every few months is enough to obtain the title. The right reason to make it deadly intersection may vary from case to case, and to fix the problem, some implementations of the appropriate remedy are required (such as introducing the pedestrian lights). This logic can be applied to the prevention of metastasis. Again, we hope to see some improvised devices or drugs to control the tumor cell traffics until they are ejected from the body.

I-c. Organ Tropism of Tumor Metastasis

Some tumor cells preferentially regrow in particular organs; breast cancer tends to metastasize to the lungs, prostate cancer cells to the bone. There may be a driving force to introduce circulating tumor cells in the more favorable distant organ. Also, matching between tumor cells and stromal cells is one of the most critical factors to determine organ tropism of the metastasis pattern (Paget's Seeds and Soil theory). It is likely that migrated tumor cells are not welcomed by the surrounding stromal cells. Tumor cells must acclimate themselves to the new environment at least to stay alive, even though they remain a dormant or an indolent state for a long time.

It is well known that some experimental cancer studies successfully extracted elements giving tumor cells propensity for metastasizing to a particular organ. For example, α-N-acetyl-neuraminyl-2,3-β-galactosyl-1,3)-N-acetylgalactosaminide α-2,6-sialyltransferase 5 (ST6GALNAC5 [17];), SPARC (secreted protein acidic and rich in cysteine [18],), IL-11 [19, 20], or claudin-2 [21] enhances preponderance of breast cancer cell metastasis in the brain, lung, bone, or liver, respectively.

I-d. Pre-metastatic Phase

As described above, it seems to be sure that some specific molecules originated from tumor cells or tumor-associated cells determine the malignancy of tumor cells. These molecular expression patterns could be used as a fingerprint to predict the possibility of future metastasis, and this can be perceived intuitively. Here, we would like to discuss the other side of the story. Stromal cells, participating in the formation of the microenvironment in metastatic site, are as important as tumor cells. Because there is organ tropism in tumor cells, there should be the same feature in the stromal cells.

Tumor-bearing mouse model system has revealed the existence of pre-metastatic niche in the remote organ before tumor cells derived from the primary tumor physically show up. Subcutaneously implanted tumor cells emit cytokine signals as it grows, and these signaling molecules are sensed by the lung endothelial or epithelial cells to trigger the inflammatory reactions including enhancement of myeloid-derived suppressor cell population and vascular permeability. These factors work together to attract the circulating tumor cells to the lungs and to protect them from the immune system. As a result, the chances of tumor metastasis are fatally augmented.

We have reported that the S100A8-Serum amyloid A3 (SAA3)-the Toll-like receptor 4 (TLR4) cascade plays crucial roles in the pre-metastatic phase in the lungs of tumor-bearing mice [22 - 24]. Our interpretation is that the S100A8-SAA3-TLR4 cascade accounts for the lung-specific metastasis. Moreover, once the pre-metastatic phase is formed, SAA3 is amplified in the resident epithelial cells in an autocrine manner [25]. A well-known inflammatory chemokine, Ccl2 is at the upstream of the cascade and responsible for hyperpermeability of the blood vessel through phosphorylation of FAK (focal adhesion kinase) to loosen endothelial cell-cell connection [26]. We also find out that the involvement of Eph-ephrin system in controlling the blood vessel permeability. Cell culture experiments demonstrate that Eph-ephrin interaction has a huge contribution to the endothelial cell-cell adhesion [27, 28]. The part of the pre-metastatic phase will be further discussed in the later section.

To our surprise, communication between a tumor and the other organ is not limited to the normal tissue. One report unraveled that one solid tumor might have a contact with the other. As one example, a mouse model study showed that a malignant tumor stimulate the bone marrow to secrete osteopontin, which in turn instigated growth of otherwise-indolent tumor apart from the original malignant tumor [9]. The report indicates that a tumor with multiple nodules is more adamant than solitary tumor because they are somewhat resonating each other.

II. CANCER STEM CELL, RECENT PROGRESS

Shortly after emerging in the field of cancer study, the concept of cancer stem cells became prevalent. There are myriad of original and reviewing papers inundating in top rated journals. Thanks to the rapidly growing research field, the contents are updated fairly frequently so that researchers have to renew the knowledge very often to keep up on the front line [29 - 38].

II-a. Definition of Cancer Stem Cell

Based on the analogy with the normal stem cell, cancer stem cell is expected to have two main properties, self-renewal, and differentiation. However, there are huge differences between normal and cancer stem cell in some aspects. In the case of normal stem cell, differentiation confers cells to specific functions to be a component of an organ. On the contrary, cancer stem cells randomly generate tumor cells with no apparent order in the tumor. Furthermore, cancer stem cells are expected to have their character such as chemoresistance, although it is not considered to be a prerequisite for the definition of cancer stem cell.

A classical DNA alkylating agent, Temozolomide, abolished proliferating tumor cells but not quiescent cells. This result indicates that Temozolomide did not eradicate tumor because cancer stem cells were refractory to it, although initial responses for the Temozolomide treatment seemed to be excellent. The reagent destructed proliferating tumor cells to shrink the tumor mass. After the certain period of Temozolomide treatment in glioblastoma model mouse, however, Temozolomide resistant cells regained its population to start regrowth of the tumor [39].

II-b. Metastatic Stem Cell

The metastatic stem cell is proposed by Massagué and co-workers [35]. The metastatic stem cell is not equal to the disseminated tumor cell but is expected to be a small portion of the tumor cells because various types of tumor cells and tumor-associated stromal cells can spread from the primary tumor site. It is highly like that metastatic stem cells already exist before its dissemination, but further investigations are needed for their detailed characterization. At least, metastatic stem cells should have an ability to initiate tumor re-growth in a distant organ, but not necessarily hold chemoresistance or cell markers peculiar to cancer stem cells.

II-c. Cancer Stem Cell and Markers

Flow cytometry is a very powerful technique to isolate and characterize the cancer stem cells. Today, many researchers rely on molecules expressed on the cell surface for the identification. A high-throughput flow cytometry screening, in which CD321 (JAM-A), CD63 (a tetraspanin family member), CD87 (urokinase receptor), CD49e (integrin α5), CD26 (dipeptidyl peptidase-4), CD54 (intracellular adhesion molecule-1; ICAM-1), CD29 (integrin β1), CD44 (a hyaluronic acid receptor), and CD49f (integrin α6) were used, was carried out to separate a self-renewal cell group from glioblastoma. Among them, JAM-A was found to be characteristic of the cancer stem cells [40]. Authors confirmed that JAM-A blocking antibody or gene knockdown did not only decrease their self-renewal and adhesion but also increased their apoptosis. JAM-A is dispensable for normal neural stem/progenitor cells. Other molecules, CD24 (a sialoglycoprotein) and CD133 (prominin-1) have been used as a marker to identify cancer stem cells.

It should be noted that, however, there is an objection claiming that even the group identified by the surface molecule expression pattern is mixed populations in terms of genomic alterations [31]. Moreover, there has been no universal cancer stem cell marker for any cancer type. It is likely that multiple cancer stem cell pools within individual tumors [34]. Therefore, it indicates importance for investigations of the gene expression profile in every single cell. The gene expression pattern provides characteristic phenotype of the cells.

II-d. Cancer Stem Cells and EMT (Epithelial-mesenchymal Transition)

Recent studies concluded that the concept of the cancer stem cell is closely related to EMT. Phenotypic plasticity of cancer stem-like properties is mediated by TGF-β, PDGF (platelet-derived growth factor), IL-6, and Wnt signaling. EMT is a critical event for tumor cells to embark on metastasis. In order to start an invasion into surrounding tissues and to accomplish metastasis procedures until beginning of the tumor regrowth, tumor cells must change their morphology from an epithelial cell form to a mesenchymal cell form. At that moment, a chain of transcription factors works together to reconstruct the entire gene expression patterns. Twist, Snail, Slug, and Zeb are responsible transcription factors for such a dramatic change, which induce a decrease of E-cadherin, an epithelial marker, and an increase of vimentin, a mesenchymal marker, are observed during the process.

A recent new finding demonstrated that Slug and Sox9 determined the mammary stem cell state. Overexpression of Slug in luminal progenitor cells or simultaneous overexpression of Slug and Sox9 in differentiated luminal cells generated mammary stem cells. Sox9 was required for maintaining tumorigenicity [41].

Id1, inhibitor of DNA binding 1, one of the EMT related transcription factors, induced tumor-initiating properties. Id1 protein pushed back EMT process by competing against Twist1; cells highly express Id1 returned to the epithelial character, which is designated as mesenchymal to epithelial transition (MET). This step is necessary for tumor cells to restart growth as a metastatic tumor in a distant location. TGF-β repressed Id1 in normal epithelial cells but induced in breast cancer cells. Smad3/Smad4, CBP/p300, or Id3 did not revert to Snail-induced EMT. Id3 opposed EMT driven by Twist in a metastatic site [42].

There was an attempt to make a direct link between the metabolic gene expression profile and EMT. Based on quantifications of metabolic gene expression levels in cancer cell lines, remarkably upregulated 44 genes were identified and designated as a mesenchymal metabolic signature. Among them, dihydropyrimidine dehydrogenase (DPYD) was essential for EMT, but not for proliferation. Additionally, the full enzymatic activity of DPYD was required for EMT although its link with EMT is not entirely explained [43].

II-e. Tumor Heterogeneity

Genetic or epigenetic alterations accumulate during cancer progression. It has been suggested that these alterations occur either in the primary tumor formation or metastatic tumor regrowth phase or both. For instance, copy number amplifications of the genome region (4q21) which covers pro-tumor CXCL1/2 chemokine genes, were observed in tumor cells [44]. Intringuingly, one prominent ImmunoFISH analysis revealed that genetic diversity at the single cell level existed in primary tumor sites, and metastatic tumors hold a higher degree of diversity [45]. It is attributed to non-cell-autonomous driving of tumor growth. In other words, tumor growth is driven by minor tumor cell subpopulations, or by enhancing proliferation of other sub-types of cells within the tumor [46].

Epigenetic changes are also significant. Along with DNA methylation, polycomb repressor-mediated silencing at H3K27me3 keeps transcription factors from binding to the promoter region. It has been known that H3K4, H3K9, H3K27 are involved in epigenetic regulations. H3K4 and H3K9 methylation triggers the initiation of transcription. Histone acetylation promotes transcription, whereas histone deacetylase and lysine specific demethylase (LSD1) on H3K9me3 repress transcription. Relationships between epigenetic changes and tumor malignancy can be found everywhere in today's cancer research reports.

A laboratory mouse study clearly demonstrated that mammary cells lacking oncogenic transgenes were long-term residence in the lungs without forming ectopic tumors [47]. Differentiations of single–cell clones in liver cancer stem cells were displayed. The cells were differentiated in melanoma, lymphoma, or prostate cancer by keeping these cells in a conditioned medium [48]. Furthermore, the clinical research displayed that breast cancer cells could disseminate systemically from ductal carcinoma *in situ*, before becoming a decisively malignant tumor [49]. One excellent paper, published recently, showed a clear correlation between tumorigenicity and particular genetic alterations. Based on the survey of gene mutations and expressions in clinical and experimental samples, a zinc finger protein RBM47 was found to stabilize DKK1 mRNA to suppress tumor progression [50].

III. CANCER STEM CELL MODELS

III-a. Clonal Evolution Model

Tumor cells acquire genetic or epigenetic changes tunes the cellular phenotype. Because selection pressure is built by surrounding tissues (hypoxia, nutrition, cytokines, immune response), the cells that can afford to grow in this environment will take over the tumor. Cancer stem cells constitute a part of it.

III-b. Classical Cancer Stem Cell Model

Cancer stem cells execute self-renewal propagations and unidirectional conversions from cancer stem cell to non-cancer stem cell. In this model, the behavior of cancer stem cell is similar to that of native stem cell.

III-c. Plastic Cancer Stem Cell Model

This model is unique to cancer stem cells. Along with the above mentioned cancer stem cell self-renewal and conversion from cancer stem cell to non-cancer stem cell, retro-directional conversion from non-cancer stem cell to cancer stem cell occurs to recreate a cancer stem cell from a cancer stem cell-free subgroup. This process has been suggested to be closely related to EMT since transcription factors involved in EMT played pivotal roles in conferring tumor cells genomic plasticity.

III-d. Cancer Stem Cells From Non-cancer Stem Cells

It has been proposed that PKCα be attributed to the generation of cancer stem cells from non-cancer stem cells. PKCα activation resulted in activation of Fra1, which was a target molecule of Twist and Snail when cells were in EMT. Activated Fra1, complied with c-Jun, replaced JunB/D and c-Fos on the AP-1 binding site. In non-cancer stem cells, EGF/EGFR signaling system was working, but once it was switched to PDGF-C/PDGFR, subsequent intracellular signalings started to choose the PKCα pathway, resulting in the conversion of non-cancer stem cell to cancer stem cell [51].

The bivalent chromatin state in the cancer stem cell has been highlighted recently to account for the stemness of cancer stem cells. This idea was first introduced in normal or neoplastic cells and later applied to carcinoma cells [52]. In a breast cancer stem cell, zeb1 promoter turned out to be a bivalent chromatin state, which was characteristic of permissive H3K4me3 and restrictive H3K27me3. The mixture of the epigenetic state was considered to be an intermediate state, so called poised position, which resulted in cellular plasticity [53].

IV. CANCER STEM CELL AND PRE-METASTATIC NICHE

Interactions between cancer cells and stromal cells are vital. In the case of the normal stem cells, stem cells are found in a particular location designated as the stem cell niche, and cells in the vicinity provide signaling molecules or other conditions to maintain its stemness. Very recently, stem cell niche of the ovarian surface epithelium hilum region in the mouse ovary was identified. Hilum cells showed preferential transformation after conditional Trp53 and Rb1 inactivation [54].

In a distant organ in the pre-metastatic phase, ECM remodeling, immunosuppression, inflammation, and vascular hyperpermeability occur before tumor cell dissemination. The pre-metastatic niche can be realized upon the following four factors; secretion of cytokines and growth factors mediated by the primary tumor, hypoxia within the primary tumor, secretion of exosomes from the primary tumor, and, reduced immune surveillance [55]. As the primary tumor-derived factors, VEGF, PlGF, TNFα, TGF-β, lysyl oxidase (LOX), versican, and G-CSF were identified. Some influence in the distant organs, others do in the bone marrow. Recruitment of BMDC in distant organs preceded tumor cell migrations. Granulocytic MDSC generated ROS to suppress CD8 positive T cells, whereas monocytic MDSC produced, Arginase-1, iNOS, and ROS, to suppress lymphocyte activation. Overall, the granulocytic MDSCs are less immunosuppressive than the monocytic MDSCs. At the same time, activation of fibroblast occurs to produce fibronectin and the secretion of MMP-9 [56].

As shown in the research of molecular mechanism in tumor cells, extracting one key protein in the pre-metastatic niche formation to demonstrate its importance by using gene knockdown technique is also applicable. A recent study found that pre-metastatic niche was $P2Y_2R$ (G protein-coupled purinergic receptor) dependent. $P2Y_2R$ was responsible for HIF1α induction and LOX secretion, followed by collagen crosslinking. BMDC recruitment was also inhibited upon knockdown of $P2Y_2R$ [57].

As mentioned in the previous section, we would like to emphasize that the pre-metastatic niche is as important as migrating tumor cells. The definition of the criteria is that circulating tumor cells are malignant enough to initiate a metastatic nodule, but at the same time stromal cells accommodating them should be cooperative enough. Here, we contemplate that continuous low-level inflammatory reactions become a good impetus for the maintenance of cancer stem cells. Again, the pre-metastatic phase is produced *via* the S100A8-SAA--TLR4 cascade, and this is indispensable with the lung metastasis. We would like to look at a crosstalk with the S100A8-SAA3-TLR4 cascade in the cancer stem cell niche. TLR4 is a central molecule for innate immune responses. Not to mention that invasions of pathogens are sensed by this receptor, and instantly trigger the downstream reactions, including inflammatory cytokine expressions and myeloid derived cell recruitments. Despite the wide repertoires of TLR4, there are a few reports describing a direct relationship between TLR4 and the cancer stem cell [58]. A renowned stem cell related molecule, Nanog was at the downstream of TLR4 signaling to maintain the stemness of tumor cells. We consider that endogenous ligands are more suitable as the stimulant of the TLR4-Nanog axis than LPS because in the tumor microenvironment there might be affluent TLR4 endogenous ligands, although the authors did not specify that whether Nanog was upregulated upon stimulation of TLR4 with an endogenous ligand instead of LPS.

Given the fact that many molecules have been added to the line-up of endogenous TLR4 ligand, it is not surprising to see some endogenous ligands have a certain role in cancer stem cell biology. Further investigations are expected to expose a hidden role of the TLR4-endogenous ligand signaling. To distinguish from the reactions exerted by unwanted endotoxin contamination, biochemical analysis of TLR4/MD-2-endogenous ligands with high purity must be guaranteed before going into further biological assays. So far, other than S100A8 and SAA3, biglycan, decorin, and HMGB1 meet the criteria to be an endogenous agonist for TLR4 and its binding partner MD-2. Biochemical studies of these four proteins determined binding constants against TLR4/MD-2. Biglycan was upregulated to remodel their structures in the tumor endothelial cells [59]. In this chapter, we would like to show our data to show potential binding structures of the biglycan-TLR4/MD-2 complex in Fig. (**2**). These five structures are determined by a computational simulation known as CyClus [60]. We have reported the same docking simulations of HMGB1-TLR4/MD-2 [61] and S100A8-TLR4/MD-2 [62]. It should be noted that bottom three structures are completely different from formerly reported structures. In the structures, biglycan protein (red chain in Fig. **2**) comes in the center hole of TLR4 (blue chain) and has only a few contacts with MD-2 (green chain). The HMGB1 and S100A8 binding styles are similar to the top two structures shown in Fig. (**2**). Ligand molecule binds on the outer surface of TLR4 and MD-2. The computational simulation results of biglycan-TLR4/M--2 imply that biglycan might have a unique binding style to TLR4/MD-2. This fact can be interpreted that there might be of biological importance in the biglycan-TLR4/MD-2 interactions. Since decorin shares its basic structure with biglycan, decorin is also expected to have very similar binding structures to biglycan in the complex with TLR4/MD-2. Decorin controlled inflammation and tumor growth through upregulation of pro-inflammatory molecules, PDCD4 (Programmed cell death 4) and miR-21 in macrophages [63]. HMGB1 was also shown to be a critical molecule in the lung metastasis of B16 tumor-bearing mice model study. Non-infectious inflammation induced by ultraviolet irradiation independently recruited myeloid derived suppressor cells to the tumor site and accelerated tumor cell invasions [65]. S100A4 was reported to be a potential TLR4/MD-2 endogenous ligand, with a direct correlation with upregulation of both SAA1 and SAA3. In the publication, there was no statement on the endotoxin level of S100A4 used in the experiments [66]. However, S100A4 was possible to form a heterodimer complex with S100A9 to bind TLR4/MD-2, and the heterodimer complex formation was enhanced in the presence of Zn^{2+} [67]. Other proteins, including peroxiredoxin, resistin, surfactant proteins, Fetuin A, and HMGN1, are putative candidates to be a TLR4/MD-2 endogenous ligand. Except for surfactant proteins, these proteins were reported to be an agonist, and they surfaced from animal studies or cell biological studies. These studies guaranteed that proteins in question were eligible to stimulate the TLR4/MD-2 system but did not exemplify their direct interactions with TLR4/MD-2. Table **1** summarizes exogenous and endogenous ligands for TLRs.

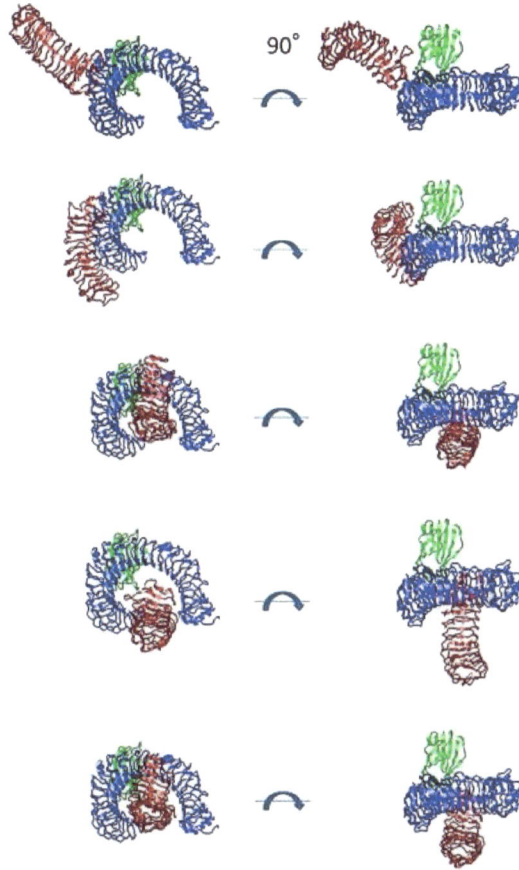

Fig. (2). Five model structures of biglycan-TLR4/MD-2 determined by the computational simulation. The left five structures present the side view of the complexes, and the 90° rotation of each complex (top view) are shown on the right. Structural data for TLR4 (blue) and MD-2 (green) is taken from PDB: 2Z64 and data for biglycan (red) is obtained from PDB: 2FT3. In this legend, PDB: 2Z64 and 2FT3 represent the identification numbers for each structure given by the Protein Data Bank (PDB). Courtesy of Drs. Takemura and Kitao (Institute of Molecular and Cellular Biosciences, The University of Tokyo).

Apart from the lung pre-metastatic niche, different organs such as bone may form different types of pre-metastatic niche. Primary prostate cancer induced abnormal formation and turnover of the bone prior to actual metastasis, although they are asymptomatic in patients. In a tumor-bearing mouse model system, platelet depletion inhibited tumor-induced bone formation. It was attributed to the sequestration of tumor-derived proteins, including MMP-1 and TGF-β [68]. Other research reported that tumor-specific T cells induced an osteolytic bone disease before colonization in the bone. *In vivo* inhibition of RANKL, a pro-osteoclastogenesis cytokine, blocked the bone metastasis [69].

Table 1. Exogenous and endogenous ligands for TLRs [64]. In the TLR4 endogenous ligands, molecules, the direct binding with TLR4/MD-2 is supported by biochemical studies, are in bold, and, it requires further biochemical confirmations, are in italics, respectively.

	Exogenous ligands	Endogenous ligands
TLR 1	Triacyl lipopeptides (Bacteria & mycobacteria)	
TLR 2	Peptidoglycan, LTA (Gram-positive bacteria), Lipoarabinomannan (Mycobacteria), Lipopeptide (mycoplasma), Zymosan, Glucuronoxylomannan, Phosphlipomannan (Fungi), Porins (Neisseria), LPS (Leptospira)	Biglycan, Carboxyalkylpyrrole, Endoplasmin, HMGB1, HSP60, HSP70, Human cardiac myosin, Hyaluronan, Monosodium urate crystals, PAUF, Versican, SNAPIN
TLR 3	Double-strand RNA (Virus)	mRNA
TLR 4	LPS (Gram-negative bacteria), Mannan (Candida albicans), Envelope proteins (RSV, MMTV), Glycoinositolphospholipids (Trypanosoma)	**Biglycan**, α-crystallin A chain, β-defensin 2, Endoplasmin (gp96), Fibrinogen, Fibronectin, Heparan sulfate, **HMGB1**, *HSP22, HSP60, HSP70, HSP72,* Hyaluronan, *Monosodium urate crystals,* OxPAPC, **PAUF, Prx1, Resistin, S100 proteins, SAA3, SP-A,** Tenascin-C, **Fetuin-A**
TLR 5	Flagellin (Bacteria)	
TLR 6	Diacyl lipopeptides (mycoplasma), Peptidoglycan (Gram-positive bacteria), Zymosan (Fungi)	Versican
TLR 7	Single strand RNA (Virus)	RNA, siRNA
TLR 8	Single strand RNA (Virus)	Human cardiac myosin, siRNA
TLR 9	Unmethylated CpG DNA (Microbes)	DNA, HMGB1, Carboxy (alkylpyrrole) protein adducts

Lymph node metastasis is also crucial. It is widely accepted that lymph node metastasis precedes distant organ metastasis so that in clinical diagnosis it is used to forecast the malignancy of tumors. In many cases, sentinel lymph nodes were removed in surgical tumor resections regardless overt metastasis in the lymph nodes, although the efficacy of lymph node dissection is still controversy. In order to investigate structural changes elicited by absorptions of tumor cells in the proximal lymph nodes or the pre-metastatic effect of distal lymph nodes, some studies focused on the difference between sentinel lymph nodes and remote lymph nodes. If all lymph nodes are created equally, their comparisons should be very good indicators to display the pre-metastatic phase. Based on comparisons of the pre-metastatic lymph nodes of esophageal cancer patients, DKK1, a Wnt pathway inhibitor, expression was significantly downregulated in the metastasis-free lymph nodes in patients with proximal lymph node metastasis [70].

V. TUMOR MICROENVIRONMENT AND CANCER STEM CELL NICHE

Most parts of the tumor are filled with non-cancer stem cells, originally differentiated from cancer stem cells, and they are the major factor to create macroscopic tumor nodules. The differentiated cancer cells have another important role to be prosperous, supporting cancer stem cell niche by providing several liquid factors. Mouse pluripotent cancer stem cells were produced by treatment with conditioned medium derived from Lewis Lung Carcinoma cells [71].

Hypoxia is one of the essential elements of the cancer stem cell niche. Gefitinib-resistant lung cancer stem cells were persistent and extremely quiescent and increased under hypoxic condition. In this condition, IGF-1 was also upregulated, and inhibition of HIF1α or IGF-1R decreased the Gefitinib resistant fractions [72]. Carbonic anhydrase, which is induced by hypoxia, played a protective role in cancer stem cells. One of the isozymes (CAIX) is correlated with poor prognosis for breast cancer metastasis, and it was required in hypoxia for the expansion and maintenance of CD44^{high}-CD24^{low} cancer stem cell population [73]. CAIX inhibition with either transfection of shRNA of chemical inhibitor (CAI017) was effectively reduced tumor size in the model systems. Additionally, CAIX inhibition combined with paclitaxel treatment significantly inhibited the tumor growth and lung metastasis [73].

Inactivation of von Hippel-Lindau tumor suppressor (VHL) mediates HIF2α degradation. Loss of VHL seemed to begin a vicious circle into tumorigenesis and metastasis. However, the relationship between VHL and tumor metastasis did not appear to be straightforward. Loss of VHL in renal cancer cells was necessary to initiate tumor formation, but not sufficient to metastasis. Additional subsequent epigenetic changes were necessary. Combination with H3K27me3 demethylation events in the CXCR4 promoter region and DNA demethylation events at cytohesin 1 interacting protein (CYTIP) followed by the VHL-loss allowed theses protein to express with high level. Finally, CXCR4 and CYTIP enhanced AP1 transcriptional responses, cell adhesion, cell migration, and support stem-cell fitness [74].

Inflammatory cytokines released from stromal cells give cancer cells enough chances to survive. Cytokines like TNFα, their levels were to be elevated in chemotherapy, stimulated tumor cells to activate the CXCL1/2 axis, which in turn activated CD11b/Gr-1 double positive myeloid cells, resulting in secretion of S100A8/A9 heterodimer to facilitate cancer cell survival [75]. Thus, the combination of doxorubicin-cyclophosphamide plus a CXCR2 antagonist, which blocks the CXCL1/2 mediated cancer cell survival, was far more effective in reducing tumor size than the conventional chemotherapy alone [75]. As one of the mechanisms, IL-1β induced prostaglandin E2 (PGE_2) in mesenchymal stem cells. Then, PGE_2 activated IL-6, IL-8, and GRO-α (growth-related oncogene) in mesenchymal stem cells in an autocrine manner. Along with these cytokines, PGE_2 bound to its cell surface receptor, EP4, expressed in cancer cells, to ignite intracellular β-catenin signaling to activate local invasion and EMT, and to enhance the stemness in the cancer cells [76]. In the case of brain tumor metastasis, IL-1β derived from tumor cells activated astrocytes to upregulate Jagged1 expression. The Jagged1 protein in the astrocytes stimulated Notch signaling in the cancer stem cells in turn, leading to the promotion of cancer stem cells self-renewal and gross tumor enlargement through upregulation of Hes5 [77].

VI. INTERACTION BETWEEN TUMOR CELLS AND STROMAL CELLS

So far, it has been known that stromal cells directly interact with tumor cells to facilitate their survival or proliferation.

VI-a. Tumor-associated Monocytes/macrophages

The tumor-associated macrophage is the most investigated species among tumor-associated stromal cells. In respect to this, a number of reports have been published so far. Macrophages are categorized two classes based on the character and gene expression pattern. Surface molecular markers can be used to distinguish a particular class of macrophages. M1 type macrophages provide anti-tumor activities, whereas M2 type macrophages promote tumor proliferation or suppress immune responses against tumor cells. IL-17 mediated communication between macrophages and tumor cells [78]. The colony stimulation factor-1 receptor (CSF-1R) inhibition changed the macrophage polarization from M2 type to M1 type to block glioma progression [79]. Tumor-associated monocyte/macrophages created the cancer stem cell niche. Direct contact of macrophages with tumor cells *via* CD11b-CD90 and Ephrin-EphA4. EphA4-PLCγ-PKCδ and Src activated IL-6 and IL-8 productions in cancer stem cells, which stimulated cancer stem cells to let them maintain stem-like status [80]. Moreover, these macrophages are reported to help tumor cells proliferate after chemotherapy [81]. Thus, the increase of such tumor-associated macrophages is recognized as a poor prognosis. CD14 positive monocytes are converted to M2 macrophage by cancer stem-like cells in chemoresistant tumors, producing macrophage colony stimulating factor (M-CSF). These cells accelerated tumor growth [82]. Ovarian CD133 positive cancer stem-like cells self-renewal was promoted by IL-17 produced by CD4 positive T cells or CD68 positive macrophages [83].

VI-b. Tumor-associated Fibroblasts

It has been known that tumor-associated fibroblasts enhanced chances of metastasis as well as tumor-associated macrophages. In the tail vein injection assay, tumor metastasis was increased when tumor cells were mixed with tumor-associated fibroblasts.

Periostin expresses in mesenchymal stem cells and promotes stem-like phenotype in breast cancer cells [84]. The triple negative breast tumor had high Src activity. The high Src activity fractions easily accomplished the bone metastasis. In the primary tumor site with high metastatic potential, insulin-like growth factor-1

(IGF-1)/CXCL12 secreted from tumor-associated fibroblasts was attributed to high Src activity of the tumor cells. *In vitro* cell culture experiments, tumor cells were confirmed to be a high Src activity, under the condition of co-culture with mesenchymal stem cells. In this case, mesenchymal stem cells were the source of IGF-1/CXCL12 [85].

VI-c. Tumor-associated Adipocytes

It is very intriguing that preadipocyte isolated from white adipose tissue injected into tumor-bearing mice *via* the tail vein showed unequivocal recruitment of the preadipocytes into the tumor. Furthermore, these preadipocytes even helped tumor growth [86]. The actual functions of preadipocytes at the tumor neighborhoods have not been elucidated.

The unique point of the tumor-associated adipocyte is that these cells supply nutrition to tumor cells so that tumor growth can be accelerated. Fatty acid binding protein 4 (FABP4) was blamed for the rapid tumor proliferation and invasion into surrounding tissues [87 - 89].

Another pivotal feature in tumor-associated adipocyte what we would like to emphasize is that differentiated adipocytes can dedifferentiate into premature cells. It has been demonstrated that a ceiling culture after isolation of adipose tissues allowed maintaining a premature cell group [90]. The cultured cells could differentiate into various types of cells under appropriate conditions. In this method, just physical tension elicited dedifferentiation potential of the cells. Thus, the same things possibly would happen in the tumor neighborhoods because growing tumor was wielding physical force to expand itself against the perimeter.

VI-d. Tumor-associated Dendritic Cells

Dendritic cells usually function as antigen-presenting cells by interacting with an exotic pathogen and T cells. Recent publications supported that tumor-associated dendritic cells are immune-suppressive and promote cancer progression in a paracrine manner. Secretions of a pro-tumor substance, resistin [91] or Galectin-1 [92] from tumor-associated dendritic cells were identified. Particularly interesting is that dendritic cells existing within or marginal area of the tumor were ingesting tumor-derived proteins constitutively and presenting tumor antigens to T cells [93]. It was mysterious that these T cells eventually failed to attack tumor cells. Tumor growth in mice with spontaneous luminal breast cancer, in which mammary tumor virus-polyoma middle T cassette was inserted, was retarded by T cell injection, but it did not last long. It was interpreted that T cells became tolerant towards tumor cells, after having contact with tumor-associated dendritic cells [93].

VI-e. Tumor-associated Neutrophils

It has been proposed that there be two types of tumor-associated neutrophil, anti-tumor N1 and pro-tumor N2, similar to the macrophage classification [94]. In an early-stage lung cancer study, tumor-associated neutrophils were shown to stimulate T cell responses, but not immune-suppressive phenotype [95, 96]. These cells seem to be N1 type neutrophils.

VI-f. Tumor-associated Natural Killer Cells

Natural killer cells constitute another subset of tumor infiltrating or tumor-associated immune cells. The entire biological behaviors of natural killer cells have not been fully understood. It has been suggested that natural killer cells are prone to be tumor progression and pro-angiogenic characters [97].

VII. DORMANT TUMOR CELLS

Dormancy is one of the top concerns in cancer diseases. It is believed that, due to the nature of dormant tumor cells, some cancer survivors come across relapse or metastasis after being sentenced remission more than a decade ago. A dormant tumor is so small, calm, and long latency period that it is somewhat difficult to detect or reproduce a model system to investigate it.

According to the descriptions in the recent publications, tumor dormancy is constituted cellular dormancy, angiogenic dormancy, and immune surveillance. Tumor cells in cellular dormancy switch cellular metabolism to a low energy consumption mode and retain cell cycle arrest state. Thus, the dormancy allows tumor cells survive in a poor condition such as a shortage of nutrients or hypoxia. Tumor cells in angiogenic dormancy do not increase in size because the lack of ability to recruit blood vessels and promote neovascularization. Immune surveillance means that the immune system suppresses the proliferation of tumor cells. It is certain that there is a selection pressure built by immune cells (neutrophil, macrophage, or dendritic cells) and surrounding normal cells to kick out pre-mature abnormal cells at the initial stages of tumor progression. Thus, there is a competition between tumor and tumor suppression factors in the microenvironment [98]. Such long-term equilibrium can maintain dormant tumor cells in a system as well as a solitary dormant tumor cell.

There are three possible strategies to brace for dormant tumor cells; 1) eradicating dormant tumor cells, 2) prolonging dormancy of the dormant tumor cells, 3) a combination of anti-proliferation plus dormancy-inducing therapy. Given the fact that dormant tumor cells are quiescent and insensitive to chemical interventions, the first option does not seem to be a good solution. We prefer the second option. Keeping dormant cells dormant without excess interventions appears to be the best way to handle them at this stage. Obviously, communications between tumor, a future metastatic site, and bone marrow turn out to be more often than people initially thought. In relation to the dormancy, tumor cells in bone marrow are surveyed for the purpose of diagnosis, although little is known about it. Clinically, observing disseminated tumor cells in the bone marrow in cancer patients is a poor prognosis. Further study unraveled that BMP7 triggered dormancy of prostate tumor cells in the bone marrow. In addition, BMP4 inhibitor COCO was found to prevent dormancy of 4T1 cells [99]. Leaving from the dormancy may require different molecules. In the case of pancreatic ductal adenocarcinoma, c-Myc upregulation was sufficient to restart cancer progression that fell a dormant state [100].

Since the tumor microenvironment has substantial contributions to determining the fate of tumor cells, it is not surprising to see its roles to control their dormancy. Fibrosis with collagen and fibronectin deposition triggered mammary tumor cells switch from a dormant to a proliferative state. The combination of a Src inhibitor (AZD0530) and an MEK1/2 inhibitor (AZD6244) delayed metastatic growth [101]. A hypoxia tolerant pancreatic cancer cell line AsPC-1 entered a dormant state in chronic hypoxia. In this state, AKT phosphorylation was reduced. On the contrary, forced activation of AKT in this cell line resulted in undergoing proliferation state and not hypoxia tolerant any longer [102].

VIII. CIRCULATING TUMOR CELLS

Detecting and analyzing circulating tumor cells is the most hopeful early diagnosis. Enumerating tumor cells in 10-20 ml of blood taken from patient allows us to predict their future outcomes or to monitor the efficacy of treatments. First of all, analysis of circulating tumor cells does not ask patients tough burdens. Second, this method, also known as 'liquid biopsy', is so sensitive that can detect the onset of cancer earlier than other conventional detection methods. A recent COPD patients study revealed that infusion of tumor cells in the blood vessel, so-called 'Sentinel circulating tumor cells' preceded a development of tangible, solid tumor in the lungs [103].

Numbers of circulating tumor cells may vary patient to patient. Usually, 1-10 cells were observed in 1 ml of patient blood while no cells in blood taken from healthy donors. In some cases, the number exceeded 100 per 1 ml blood. Moreover, the tumor cell number implies a poor prognosis. In other words, the more circulating tumor cells exist, the less progression-free survival period is expected. Of course, the tumor-initiating ability of the circulating cell is another important factor. Circulating tumor DNA is also used in diagnosis. A DNA fragment containing mutations, such as TP53 mutations, was reported to have a correlation with tumorigenesis or tumor progression. DNA fragments purified from plasma can be subjected to this analysis. The amount of circulating tumor DNA did not show any correlation with patient outcomes, but it was useful to decide strategy of tumor treatments because such mutations sensitively reflected the type of the tumor in question [104, 105].

In many cases, characters of circulating tumor cells are somewhat different from that of the primary tumor. In the paper of Haber and co-workers, based on the gene expression profiling, three types of circulating tumor cells were defined; classical CTC, platelet adhered CTC and proliferative CTC [Ting *et al.*, 2014]. Platelet-adhered CTC expressed platelet markers CD41 and CD61, whereas proliferative CTC had a prominent cellular proliferative signature. The majority of circulating tumor cells was classical CTC, demonstrating loss of epithelial markers (E-cadherin and MUC1) and enrichment of a stem cell marker, Aldh1a1. Comparison of gene expression patterns between primary tumor (mouse pancreatic ductal adenocarcinoma) and circulating tumor cells revealed that three extracellular matrix genes (Decorin, KLF4, IGFBP5) were remarkably upregulated in classical CTCs [106].

Considering the origin of circulating tumor cells, two types of tumor cells may exist in the bloodstream. One is an epithelial cell phenotype, holding epithelial cell adhesion molecule (EpCAM) expression. This type of cells are supposed to be pushed out passively (Passive intravasation). The other type is a mesenchymal phenotype due to EMT in the primary tumor site, having an invasion activity to attain intravasation by oneself alone (Active intravasation). These facts indicate that the circulating tumor cell is heterogeneous and not always EpCAM positive. According to the circulating tumor cell detection system, provided images clearly showed that the majority of the cells were single cells, but clusters did also exist. Tumor cell clusters and the stromal cells (such as tumor-associated macrophages) are also possible because there are many immune cells, probably the tumor-friendly type of cells around the primary tumor. The tumor cell clusters were constituted of 2-50 tumor cells [107]. Clustered tumor cells are more likely to survive so that the metastasis rate of the clustered tumor cells is higher than that of single tumor cells.

There are two types of the detection system, label-dependent and label-independent method. In the label dependent circulating tumor cell enrichment, EpCAM/or MUC1 expressing cells are captured. For instance, FDA approved CellSearch equips magnetic beads coated with anti-EpCAM. Its capture rates are estimated roughly 70-80%, depending on tumor type. Pre-treatment with anti-CD45 coated magnetic beads as a negative depletion step may be applied to enhance the processing speed, recovery rate and purity of tumor cells. In the label-independent enrichment, cells are fractionated based on their physical properties, such as density, size, invasive capacity, or surface charge. By using these devices, circulating tumor cells initially scattered at the ratio of one in 10^6-10^8 blood cells was enriched to be one in 10^2-10^3 blood cells. Isolated circulating tumor cells were subjected to further analysis, including PCR and protein secretion [108].

Can circulating tumor cells make pre-metastatic niche at distant organs? Probably yes. These cells can secrete inflammatory cytokines, which are necessary to prepare the pre-metastatic niche in distant organs, as shown in a single cell analysis [109]. Even though circulating tumor cells are very rare, the signal might be intensified by tumor-associated cells or tumor cell-tumor cell communications because the secreted proteins in the blood vessel were efficiently conveyed to the organ.

IX. RESHAPING PRE-METASTATIC NICHE MODELS

Inflammatory reactions are not constant; it should be an oscillation style because there are multiple negative feedback systems to contain generations of an excess amount of cytokines. For instance, IL-8 is regulated very tightly at mRNA and protein levels. TNFα stimulation quickly upregulates IL-8 transcription and translation to secrete IL-8, but at the same time, produced IL-8 conducts repression of its transcription and translation. NF-κB oscillation is one of the most intensely studied model cases [110]. In this model, NF-κB is set to be a key transcription factor for IL-8 expression. NF-κB forms a complex with IκBα in the cytosol, and this complex is the inactivated form. Once IκBα is phosphorylated, IκBα detaches from NF-κB followed by receiving phosphorylation to be the active form and translocating into nuclei. A computational approach re-defined these intriguing intracellular signaling pathways to find out that the NF-κB oscillation was controlled by three factors; amounts of NF-κB, IκBα, and IκBα mRNA [111].

Endothelial cell-cell contacts are loosened where inflammatory reactions occur. The Evans blue injection assay visualized such high permeability regions in the lungs and interestingly such lungs in pre-metastatic phase exhibited a patchy pattern, a mixture of high and low permeability regions. The pattern is expected to change due to the oscillation of inflammatory reactions, although we only have endpoint data. The tumor cell homing assay indicated that tumor cell extravasation occurs at the high permeability region.

It is reported that approximately 3% of metastatic carcinoma were diagnosed with unknown primary cancer. The site of origin was widely spread, and individual treatments were necessary after analyzing the phenotype of the metastatic carcinoma, including gene mutations and molecular markers [112]. The common features of metastatic carcinomas are rapid progression and dissemination so that tumor cells, even after leaving the primary site grow faster than the remnants at the primary site. It may be possible that progressions of the primary tumor were totally retarded by the host defense system or lack of proper support. Alternatively, the location of the primary site was too easy to access to the blood vessel. Recently, the usefulness of ^{18}F-fluorodeoxyglucose PET-CT was reported. This technique successfully identified primary tumor locations in 39% of the patients with extracervical cancer of unknown primary site [113]. These primary site tumors were so small that conventional methods were not able to detect. Whether the primary tumor had a contribution to facilitating metastasis by forming a pre-metastatic niche is a big question.

X. CONCLUSION

For those who are engaged in the field of cancer study, the ultimate goal is to get over cancer. Even we feel as if we are about to wade into a quagmire and are at only the beginning. One of the most impressive findings of the recent studies is the conversion of non-cancer stem cells to cancer stem cells. It makes the cancer stem cell evasive, and numbers of breakthrough are needed to understand it thoroughly. Nonetheless, technology never stops making progress. Every time new concept, new reagents, or new devices are introduced in the field, we will come across new features of cancer. With no concrete evidence, we think that TLR4/MD-2 endogenous ligands will rescue the predicament. We continue our ongoing TLR4/MD-2 endogenous ligand investigations, hoping to make a huge difference in the future.

CONFLICT OF INTEREST

The authors confirm that they have no conflict of interest to declare for this publication.

ACKNOWLEDGEMENTS

The authors would like to thank Drs. Kitao and Takemura (Institute of Molecular and Cellular Biosciences, The University of Tokyo) for providing the docking simulation data.

REFERENCES

[1]   Gocheva V, Wang HW, Gadea BB, *et al.* IL-4 induces cathepsin protease activity in tumor-associated macrophages to promote cancer growth and invasion. Genes Dev 2010; 24(3): 241-55.
[http://dx.doi.org/10.1101/gad.1874010] [PMID: 20080943]

[2]   Bitu CC, Kauppila JH, Bufalino A, *et al.* Cathepsin K is present in invasive oral tongue squamous cell carcinoma *in vivo* and *in vitro*. PLoS One 2013; 8(8): e70925.
[http://dx.doi.org/10.1371/journal.pone.0070925] [PMID: 23951042]

[3]   DeNardo DG, Barreto JB, Andreu P, *et al.* CD4(+) T cells regulate pulmonary metastasis of mammary carcinomas by enhancing protumor properties of macrophages. Cancer Cell 2009; 16(2): 91-102.
[http://dx.doi.org/10.1016/j.ccr.2009.06.018] [PMID: 19647220]

[4]   Wyckoff JB, Wang Y, Lin EY, *et al.* Direct visualization of macrophage-assisted tumor cell intravasation in mammary tumors. Cancer Res 2007; 67(6): 2649-56.
[http://dx.doi.org/10.1158/0008-5472.CAN-06-1823] [PMID: 17363585]

[5]   Heidemann F, Schildt A, Schmid K, *et al.* Selectins mediate small cell lung cancer systemic metastasis. PLoS One 2014; 9(4): e92327.
[http://dx.doi.org/10.1371/journal.pone.0092327] [PMID: 24699516]

[6]   Brown DM, Ruoslahti E. Metadherin, a cell surface protein in breast tumors that mediates lung metastasis. Cancer Cell 2004; 5(4): 365-74.
[http://dx.doi.org/10.1016/S1535-6108(04)00079-0] [PMID: 15093543]

[7]   Padua D, Zhang XH, Wang Q, *et al.* TGFbeta primes breast tumors for lung metastasis seeding through angiopoietin-like 4. Cell 2008; 133(1): 66-77.
[http://dx.doi.org/10.1016/j.cell.2008.01.046] [PMID: 18394990]

[8]   Tang CH, Tan TW, Fu WM, Yang RS. Involvement of matrix metalloproteinase-9 in stromal cell-derived factor-1/CXCR4 pathway of lung cancer metastasis. Carcinogenesis 2008; 29(1): 35-43.
[http://dx.doi.org/10.1093/carcin/bgm220] [PMID: 17916907]

[9]   McAllister SS, Gifford AM, Greiner AL, *et al.* Systemic endocrine instigation of indolent tumor growth requires osteopontin. Cell 2008; 133(6): 994-1005.
[http://dx.doi.org/10.1016/j.cell.2008.04.045] [PMID: 18555776]

[10]   Chen Q, Zhang XH, Massagué J. Macrophage binding to receptor VCAM-1 transmits survival signals in breast cancer cells that invade the lungs. Cancer Cell 2011; 20(4): 538-49.
[http://dx.doi.org/10.1016/j.ccr.2011.08.025] [PMID: 22014578]

[11]   Chen Q, Massagué J. Molecular pathways: VCAM-1 as a potential therapeutic target in metastasis. Clin Cancer Res 2012; 18(20): 5520-5.
[http://dx.doi.org/10.1158/1078-0432.CCR-11-2904] [PMID: 22879387]

[12]   Morales M, Arenas EJ, Urosevic J, *et al.* RARRES3 suppresses breast cancer lung metastasis by regulating adhesion and differentiation. EMBO Mol Med 2014; 6(7): 865-81.
[http://dx.doi.org/10.15252/emmm.201303675] [PMID: 24867881]

[13]   Watnick RS, Rodriguez RK, Wang S, *et al.* Thrombospondin-1 repression is mediated *via* distinct mechanisms in fibroblasts and epithelial cells. Oncogene 2014.
[http://dx.doi.org/10.1038/onc.2014.228] [PMID: 25109329]

[14]   Sevenich L, Bowman RL, Mason SD, *et al.* Analysis of tumour- and stroma-supplied proteolytic networks reveals a brain-metastasis-promoting role for cathepsin S. Nat Cell Biol 2014; 16(9): 876-88.
[http://dx.doi.org/10.1038/ncb3011] [PMID: 25086747]

[15]   Shibue T, Brooks MW, Inan MF, Reinhardt F, Weinberg RA. The outgrowth of micrometastases is enabled by the formation of filopodium-like protrusions. Cancer Discov 2012; 2(8): 706-21.
[http://dx.doi.org/10.1158/2159-8290.CD-11-0239] [PMID: 22609699]

[16]   Shibue T, Brooks MW, Weinberg RA. An integrin-linked machinery of cytoskeletal regulation that enables experimental tumor initiation and metastatic colonization. Cancer Cell 2013; 24(4): 481-98. [Erratum in: Cancer Cell 2013; 24: 806-8].
[http://dx.doi.org/10.1016/j.ccr.2013.08.012] [PMID: 24035453]

[17]   Bos PD, Zhang XH, Nadal C, *et al.* Genes that mediate breast cancer metastasis to the brain. Nature 2009; 459(7249): 1005-9.
[http://dx.doi.org/10.1038/nature08021] [PMID: 19421193]

[18]   Minn AJ, Gupta GP, Siegel PM, *et al.* Genes that mediate breast cancer metastasis to lung. Nature 2005; 436(7050): 518-24.
[http://dx.doi.org/10.1038/nature03799] [PMID: 16049480]

[19]   Kang Y, Siegel PM, Shu W, *et al.* A multigenic program mediating breast cancer metastasis to bone. Cancer Cell 2003; 3(6): 537-49.
[http://dx.doi.org/10.1016/S1535-6108(03)00132-6] [PMID: 12842083]

[20]   Kang Y, He W, Tulley S, *et al.* Breast cancer bone metastasis mediated by the Smad tumor suppressor pathway. Proc Natl Acad Sci USA 2005; 102(39): 13909-14.
[http://dx.doi.org/10.1073/pnas.0506517102] [PMID: 16172383]

[21]   Tabariès S, Dupuy F, Dong Z, *et al.* Claudin-2 promotes breast cancer liver metastasis by facilitating tumor cell interactions with hepatocytes. Mol Cell Biol 2012; 32(15): 2979-91.
[http://dx.doi.org/10.1128/MCB.00299-12] [PMID: 22645303]

[22]   Hiratsuka S, Watanabe A, Aburatani H, Maru Y. Tumour-mediated upregulation of chemoattractants and recruitment of myeloid cells predetermines lung metastasis. Nat Cell Biol 2006; 8(12): 1369-75.
[http://dx.doi.org/10.1038/ncb1507] [PMID: 17128264]

[23]   Hiratsuka S, Watanabe A, Sakurai Y, *et al.* The S100A8-serum amyloid A3-TLR4 paracrine cascade establishes a pre-metastatic phase. Nat Cell Biol 2008; 10(11): 1349-55.
[http://dx.doi.org/10.1038/ncb1794] [PMID: 18820689]

[24]   Deguchi A, Tomita T, Omori T, *et al.* Serum amyloid A3 binds MD-2 to activate p38 and NF-κB pathways in a MyD88-dependent manner. J Immunol 2013; 191(4): 1856-64.
[http://dx.doi.org/10.4049/jimmunol.1201996] [PMID: 23858030]

[25]   Tomita T, Sakurai Y, Ishibashi S, Maru Y. Imbalance of Clara cell-mediated homeostatic inflammation is involved in lung metastasis. Oncogene 2011; 30(31): 3429-39.
[http://dx.doi.org/10.1038/onc.2011.53] [PMID: 21399660]

[26] Hiratsuka S, Ishibashi S, Tomita T, *et al.* Primary tumours modulate innate immune signalling to create pre-metastatic vascular hyperpermeability foci. Nat Commun 2013; 4: 1853.
[http://dx.doi.org/10.1038/ncomms2856] [PMID: 23673638]

[27] Ieguchi K, Omori T, Komatsu A, Tomita T, Deguchi A, Maru Y. Ephrin-A1 expression induced by S100A8 is mediated by the toll-like receptor 4. Biochem Biophys Res Commun 2013; 440(4): 623-9.
[http://dx.doi.org/10.1016/j.bbrc.2013.09.119] [PMID: 24103748]

[28] Ieguchi K, Tomita T, Omori T, *et al.* ADAM12-cleaved ephrin-A1 contributes to lung metastasis. Oncogene 2014; 33(17): 2179-90.
[http://dx.doi.org/10.1038/onc.2013.180] [PMID: 23686306]

[29] Valastyan S, Weinberg RA. Tumor metastasis: molecular insights and evolving paradigms. Cell 2011; 147(2): 275-92.
[http://dx.doi.org/10.1016/j.cell.2011.09.024] [PMID: 22000009]

[30] Shigdar S, Li Y, Bhattacharya S, *et al.* Inflammation and cancer stem cells. Cancer Lett 2014; 345(2): 271-8.
[http://dx.doi.org/10.1016/j.canlet.2013.07.031] [PMID: 23941828]

[31] Meacham CE, Morrison SJ. Tumour heterogeneity and cancer cell plasticity. Nature 2013; 501(7467): 328-37.
[http://dx.doi.org/10.1038/nature12624] [PMID: 24048065]

[32] Marjanovic ND, Weinberg RA, Chaffer CL. Cell plasticity and heterogeneity in cancer. Clin Chem 2013; 59(1): 168-79.
[http://dx.doi.org/10.1373/clinchem.2012.184655] [PMID: 23220226]

[33] Tam WL, Weinberg RA. The epigenetics of epithelial-mesenchymal plasticity in cancer. Nat Med 2013; 19(11): 1438-49.
[http://dx.doi.org/10.1038/nm.3336] [PMID: 24202396]

[34] Visvader JE, Lindeman GJ. Cancer stem cells: current status and evolving complexities. Cell Stem Cell 2012; 10(6): 717-28.
[http://dx.doi.org/10.1016/j.stem.2012.05.007] [PMID: 22704512]

[35] Oskarsson T, Batlle E, Massagué J. Metastatic stem cells: sources, niches, and vital pathways. Cell Stem Cell 2014; 14(3): 306-21.
[http://dx.doi.org/10.1016/j.stem.2014.02.002] [PMID: 24607405]

[36] Vanharanta S, Massagué J. Origins of metastatic traits. Cancer Cell 2013; 24(4): 410-21.
[http://dx.doi.org/10.1016/j.ccr.2013.09.007] [PMID: 24135279]

[37] Quail DF, Joyce JA. Microenvironmental regulation of tumor progression and metastasis. Nat Med 2013; 19(11): 1423-37.
[http://dx.doi.org/10.1038/nm.3394] [PMID: 24202395]

[38] Wan L, Pantel K, Kang Y. Tumor metastasis: moving new biological insights into the clinic. Nat Med 2013; 19(11): 1450-64.
[http://dx.doi.org/10.1038/nm.3391] [PMID: 24202397]

[39] Chen J, Li Y, Yu TS, *et al.* A restricted cell population propagates glioblastoma growth after chemotherapy. Nature 2012; 488(7412): 522-6.

[http://dx.doi.org/10.1038/nature11287] [PMID: 22854781]

[40]   Lathia JD, Li M, Sinyuk M, *et al.* High-throughput flow cytometry screening reveals a role for junctional adhesion molecule a as a cancer stem cell maintenance factor. Cell Reports 2014; 6(1): 117-29.
[http://dx.doi.org/10.1016/j.celrep.2013.11.043] [PMID: 24373972]

[41]   Guo W, Keckesova Z, Donaher JL, *et al.* Slug and Sox9 cooperatively determine the mammary stem cell state. Cell 2012; 148(5): 1015-28.
[http://dx.doi.org/10.1016/j.cell.2012.02.008] [PMID: 22385965]

[42]   Stankic M, Pavlovic S, Chin Y, *et al.* TGF-β-Id1 signaling opposes Twist1 and promotes metastatic colonization *via* a mesenchymal-to-epithelial transition. Cell Reports 2013; 5(5): 1228-42.
[http://dx.doi.org/10.1016/j.celrep.2013.11.014] [PMID: 24332369]

[43]   Shaul YD, Freinkman E, Comb WC, *et al.* Dihydropyrimidine accumulation is required for the epithelial-mesenchymal transition. Cell 2014; 158(5): 1094-109.
[http://dx.doi.org/10.1016/j.cell.2014.07.032] [PMID: 25171410]

[44]   Beroukhim R, Mermel CH, Porter D, *et al.* The landscape of somatic copy-number alteration across human cancers. Nature 2010; 463(7283): 899-905.
[http://dx.doi.org/10.1038/nature08822] [PMID: 20164920]

[45]   Almendro V, Kim HJ, Cheng YK, *et al.* Genetic and phenotypic diversity in breast tumor metastases. Cancer Res 2014; 74(5): 1338-48.
[http://dx.doi.org/10.1158/0008-5472.CAN-13-2357-T] [PMID: 24448237]

[46]   Marusyk A, Tabassum DP, Altrock PM, Almendro V, Michor F, Polyak K. Non-cell-autonomous driving of tumour growth supports sub-clonal heterogeneity. Nature 2014; 514(7520): 54-8.
[http://dx.doi.org/10.1038/nature13556] [PMID: 25079331]

[47]   Podsypanina K, Du YC, Jechlinger M, Beverly LJ, Hambardzumyan D, Varmus H. Seeding and propagation of untransformed mouse mammary cells in the lung. Science 2008; 321(5897): 1841-4.
[http://dx.doi.org/10.1126/science.1161621] [PMID: 18755941]

[48]   Liu H, Zhang W, Jia Y, *et al.* Single-cell clones of liver cancer stem cells have the potential of differentiating into different types of tumor cells. Cell Death Dis 2013; 4: e857.
[http://dx.doi.org/10.1038/cddis.2013.340] [PMID: 24136221]

[49]   Hüsemann Y, Geigl JB, Schubert F, *et al.* Systemic spread is an early step in breast cancer. Cancer Cell 2008; 13(1): 58-68.
[http://dx.doi.org/10.1016/j.ccr.2007.12.003] [PMID: 18167340]

[50]   Vanharanta S, Marney CB, Shu W, *et al.* Loss of the multifunctional RNA-binding protein RBM47 as a source of selectable metastatic traits in breast cancer. eLife 2014; 3
[http://dx.doi.org/10.7554/eLife.02734] [PMID: 24898756]

[51]   Tam WL, Lu H, Buikhuisen J, *et al.* Protein kinase C α is a central signaling node and therapeutic target for breast cancer stem cells. Cancer Cell 2013; 24(3): 347-64.
[http://dx.doi.org/10.1016/j.ccr.2013.08.005] [PMID: 24029232]

[52]   Chaffer CL, Brueckmann I, Scheel C, *et al.* Normal and neoplastic nonstem cells can spontaneously convert to a stem-like state. Proc Natl Acad Sci USA 2011; 108(19): 7950-5.

[http://dx.doi.org/10.1073/pnas.1102454108] [PMID: 21498687]

[53] Chaffer CL, Marjanovic ND, Lee T, *et al.* Poised chromatin at the ZEB1 promoter enables breast cancer cell plasticity and enhances tumorigenicity. Cell 2013; 154(1): 61-74.
[http://dx.doi.org/10.1016/j.cell.2013.06.005] [PMID: 23827675]

[54] Flesken-Nikitin A, Hwang CI, Cheng CY, Michurina TV, Enikolopov G, Nikitin AY. Ovarian surface epithelium at the junction area contains a cancer-prone stem cell niche. Nature 2013; 495(7440): 241-5.
[http://dx.doi.org/10.1038/nature11979] [PMID: 23467088]

[55] Sceneay J, Smyth MJ, Möller A. The pre-metastatic niche: finding common ground. Cancer Metastasis Rev 2013; 32(3-4): 449-64.
[http://dx.doi.org/10.1007/s10555-013-9420-1] [PMID: 23636348]

[56] Kaplan RN, Riba RD, Zacharoulis S, *et al.* VEGFR1-positive haematopoietic bone marrow progenitors initiate the pre-metastatic niche. Nature 2005; 438(7069): 820-7.
[http://dx.doi.org/10.1038/nature04186] [PMID: 16341007]

[57] Joo YN, Jin H, Eun SY, Park SW, Chang KC, Kim HJ. P2Y2R activation by nucleotides released from the highly metastatic breast cancer cell MDA-MB-231 contributes to pre-metastatic niche formation by mediating lysyl oxidase secretion, collagen crosslinking, and monocyte recruitment. Oncotarget 2014; 5(19): 9322-34.
[http://dx.doi.org/10.18632/oncotarget.2427] [PMID: 25238333]

[58] Chen CL, Tsukamoto H, Liu JC, *et al.* Reciprocal regulation by TLR4 and TGF-β in tumor-initiating stem-like cells. J Clin Invest 2013; 123(7): 2832-49.
[http://dx.doi.org/10.1172/JCI65859] [PMID: 23921128]

[59] Yamamoto K, Ohga N, Hida Y, *et al.* Biglycan is a specific marker and an autocrine angiogenic factor of tumour endothelial cells. Br J Cancer 2012; 106(6): 1214-23.
[http://dx.doi.org/10.1038/bjc.2012.59] [PMID: 22374465]

[60] Omori S, Kitao A. CyClus: a fast, comprehensive cylindrical interface approximation clustering/reranking method for rigid-body protein-protein docking decoys. Proteins 2013; 81(6): 1005-16.
[http://dx.doi.org/10.1002/prot.24252] [PMID: 23344972]

[61] Maru Y, Tomita T, Deguchi A, *et al.* Anti-inflammatory treatment for seemingly non-inflammatory disorders. Endocr Metab Immune Disord Drug Targets 2015; 15(2): 83-7.
[http://dx.doi.org/10.2174/1871530315021505221 23746] [PMID: 26004773]

[62] Deguchi A, Tomita T, Ohto U, *et al.* Eritoran inhibits S100A8-mediated TLR4/MD-2 activation and tumor growth by changing the immune microenvironment. Oncogene 2016; 35(11): 1445-56.
[http://dx.doi.org/10.1038/onc.2015.211] [PMID: 26165843]

[63] Merline R, Moreth K, Beckmann J, *et al.* Signaling by the matrix proteoglycan decorin controls inflammation and cancer through PDCD4 and MicroRNA-21. Sci Signal 2011; 4(199): ra75.
[http://dx.doi.org/10.1126/scisignal.2001868] [PMID: 22087031]

[64] Bald T, Quast T, Landsberg J, *et al.* Ultraviolet-radiation-induced inflammation promotes angiotropism and metastasis in melanoma. Nature 2014; 507(7490): 109-13.

[http://dx.doi.org/10.1038/nature13111] [PMID: 24572365]

[65]   Hansen MT, Forst B, Cremers N, *et al.* A link between inflammation and metastasis: serum amyloid A1 and A3 induce metastasis, and are targets of metastasis-inducing S100A4. Oncogene 2015; 34(4): 424-35.
[http://dx.doi.org/10.1038/onc.2013.568] [PMID: 24469032]

[66]   Yu L, Wang L, Chen S. Exogenous or endogenous Toll-like receptor ligands: which is the MVP in tumorigenesis? Cell Mol Life Sci 2012; 69(6): 935-49. [Exogenous or endogenous Toll-like receptor ligands: which is the MVP in tumorigenesis?].
[http://dx.doi.org/10.1007/s00018-011-0864-6] [PMID: 22048194]

[67]   Björk P, Källberg E, Wellmar U, *et al.* Common interactions between S100A4 and S100A9 defined by a novel chemical probe. PLoS One 2013; 8(5): e63012.
[http://dx.doi.org/10.1371/journal.pone.0063012] [PMID: 23667563]

[68]   Kerr BA, McCabe NP, Feng W, Byzova TV. Platelets govern pre-metastatic tumor communication to bone. Oncogene 2013; 32(36): 4319-24.
[http://dx.doi.org/10.1038/onc.2012.447] [PMID: 23069656]

[69]   Monteiro AC, Leal AC, Gonçalves-Silva T, *et al.* T cells induce pre-metastatic osteolytic disease and help bone metastases establishment in a mouse model of metastatic breast cancer. PLoS One 2013; 8(7): e68171.
[http://dx.doi.org/10.1371/journal.pone.0068171] [PMID: 23935856]

[70]   Otto B, Koenig AM, Tolstonog GV, *et al.* Molecular changes in pre-metastatic lymph nodes of esophageal cancer patients. PLoS One 2014; 9(7): e102552.
[http://dx.doi.org/10.1371/journal.pone.0102552] [PMID: 25048826]

[71]   Matsuda S, Yan T, Mizutani A, *et al.* Cancer stem cells maintain a hierarchy of differentiation by creating their niche. Int J Cancer 2014; 135(1): 27-36.
[http://dx.doi.org/10.1002/ijc.28648] [PMID: 24323788]

[72]   Murakami A, Takahashi F, Nurwidya F, *et al.* Hypoxia increases gefitinib-resistant lung cancer stem cells through the activation of insulin-like growth factor 1 receptor. PLoS One 2014; 9(1): e86459.
[http://dx.doi.org/10.1371/journal.pone.0086459] [PMID: 24489728]

[73]   Lock FE, McDonald PC, Lou Y, *et al.* Targeting carbonic anhydrase IX depletes breast cancer stem cells within the hypoxic niche. Oncogene 2013; 32(44): 5210-9.
[http://dx.doi.org/10.1038/onc.2012.550] [PMID: 23208505]

[74]   Vanharanta S, Shu W, Brenet F, *et al.* Epigenetic expansion of VHL-HIF signal output drives multiorgan metastasis in renal cancer. Nat Med 2013; 19(1): 50-6.
[http://dx.doi.org/10.1038/nm.3029] [PMID: 23223005]

[75]   Acharyya S, Oskarsson T, Vanharanta S, *et al.* A CXCL1 paracrine network links cancer chemoresistance and metastasis. Cell 2012; 150(1): 165-78.
[http://dx.doi.org/10.1016/j.cell.2012.04.042] [PMID: 22770218]

[76]   Li HJ, Reinhardt F, Herschman HR, Weinberg RA. Cancer-stimulated mesenchymal stem cells create a carcinoma stem cell niche *via* prostaglandin E2 signaling. Cancer Discov 2012; 2(9): 840-55.
[http://dx.doi.org/10.1158/2159-8290.CD-12-0101] [PMID: 22763855]

[77] Xing F, Kobayashi A, Okuda H, *et al.* Reactive astrocytes promote the metastatic growth of breast cancer stem-like cells by activating Notch signalling in brain. EMBO Mol Med 2013; 5(3): 384-96.
[http://dx.doi.org/10.1002/emmm.201201623] [PMID: 23495140]

[78] Chung AS, Wu X, Zhuang G, *et al.* An interleukin-17-mediated paracrine network promotes tumor resistance to anti-angiogenic therapy. Nat Med 2013; 19(9): 1114-23.
[http://dx.doi.org/10.1038/nm.3291] [PMID: 23913124]

[79] Pyonteck SM, Akkari L, Schuhmacher AJ, *et al.* CSF-1R inhibition alters macrophage polarization and blocks glioma progression. Nat Med 2013; 19(10): 1264-72.
[http://dx.doi.org/10.1038/nm.3337] [PMID: 24056773]

[80] Lu H, Clauser KR, Tam WL, *et al.* A breast cancer stem cell niche supported by juxtacrine signalling from monocytes and macrophages. Nat Cell Biol 2014; 16(11): 1105-17.
[http://dx.doi.org/10.1038/ncb3041] [PMID: 25266422]

[81] Lu-Emerson C, Snuderl M, Kirkpatrick ND, *et al.* Increase in tumor-associated macrophages after antiangiogenic therapy is associated with poor survival among patients with recurrent glioblastoma. Neuro-oncol 2013; 15(8): 1079-87.
[http://dx.doi.org/10.1093/neuonc/not082] [PMID: 23828240]

[82] Yamashina T, Baghdadi M, Yoneda A, *et al.* Cancer stem-like cells derived from chemoresistant tumors have a unique capacity to prime tumorigenic myeloid cells. Cancer Res 2014; 74(10): 2698-709.
[http://dx.doi.org/10.1158/0008-5472.CAN-13-2169] [PMID: 24638980]

[83] Xiang T, Long H, He L, *et al.* Interleukin-17 produced by tumor microenvironment promotes self-renewal of CD133+ cancer stem-like cells in ovarian cancer. Oncogene 2015; 34(2): 165-76.
[http://dx.doi.org/10.1038/onc.2013.537] [PMID: 24362529]

[84] Wang X, Liu J, Wang Z, *et al.* Periostin contributes to the acquisition of multipotent stem cell-like properties in human mammary epithelial cells and breast cancer cells. PLoS One 2013; 8(8): e72962.
[http://dx.doi.org/10.1371/journal.pone.0072962] [PMID: 24009721]

[85] Zhang XH, Jin X, Malladi S, *et al.* Selection of bone metastasis seeds by mesenchymal signals in the primary tumor stroma. Cell 2013; 154(5): 1060-73.
[http://dx.doi.org/10.1016/j.cell.2013.07.036] [PMID: 23993096]

[86] Zhang Y, Daquinag A, Traktuev DO, *et al.* White adipose tissue cells are recruited by experimental tumors and promote cancer progression in mouse models. Cancer Res 2009; 69(12): 5259-66.
[http://dx.doi.org/10.1158/0008-5472.CAN-08-3444] [PMID: 19491274]

[87] Nieman KM, Kenny HA, Penicka CV, *et al.* Adipocytes promote ovarian cancer metastasis and provide energy for rapid tumor growth. Nat Med 2011; 17(11): 1498-503.
[http://dx.doi.org/10.1038/nm.2492] [PMID: 22037646]

[88] Dirat B, Bochet L, Dabek M, *et al.* Cancer-associated adipocytes exhibit an activated phenotype and contribute to breast cancer invasion. Cancer Res 2011; 71(7): 2455-65.
[http://dx.doi.org/10.1158/0008-5472.CAN-10-3323] [PMID: 21459803]

[89] Herroon MK, Rajagurubandara E, Hardaway AL, *et al.* Bone marrow adipocytes promote tumor growth in bone *via* FABP4-dependent mechanisms. Oncotarget 2013; 4(11): 2108-23.

[http://dx.doi.org/10.18632/oncotarget.1482] [PMID: 24240026]

[90]   Nobusue H, Endo T, Kano K. Establishment of a preadipocyte cell line derived from mature adipocytes of GFP transgenic mice and formation of adipose tissue. Cell Tissue Res 2008; 332(3): 435-46.
[http://dx.doi.org/10.1007/s00441-008-0593-9] [PMID: 18386066]

[91]   Kuo CH, Chen KF, Chou SH, *et al.* Lung tumor-associated dendritic cell-derived resistin promoted cancer progression by increasing Wolf-Hirschhorn syndrome candidate 1/Twist pathway. Carcinogenesis 2013; 34(11): 2600-9.
[http://dx.doi.org/10.1093/carcin/bgt281] [PMID: 23955539]

[92]   Kuo PL, Huang MS, Cheng DE, Hung JY, Yang CJ, Chou SH. Lung cancer-derived galectin-1 enhances tumorigenic potentiation of tumor-associated dendritic cells by expressing heparin-binding EGF-like growth factor. J Biol Chem 2012; 287(13): 9753-64.
[http://dx.doi.org/10.1074/jbc.M111.321190] [PMID: 22291012]

[93]   Engelhardt JJ, Boldajipour B, Beemiller P, *et al.* Marginating dendritic cells of the tumor microenvironment cross-present tumor antigens and stably engage tumor-specific T cells. Cancer Cell 2012; 21(3): 402-17.
[http://dx.doi.org/10.1016/j.ccr.2012.01.008] [PMID: 22439936]

[94]   Fridlender ZG, Sun J, Kim S, *et al.* Polarization of tumor-associated neutrophil phenotype by TGF-beta: "N1" *versus* "N2" TAN. Cancer Cell 2009; 16(3): 183-94.
[http://dx.doi.org/10.1016/j.ccr.2009.06.017] [PMID: 19732719]

[95]   Granot Z, Henke E, Comen EA, King TA, Norton L, Benezra R. Tumor entrained neutrophils inhibit seeding in the premetastatic lung. Cancer Cell 2011; 20(3): 300-14.
[http://dx.doi.org/10.1016/j.ccr.2011.08.012] [PMID: 21907922]

[96]   Eruslanov EB, Bhojnagarwala PS, Quatromoni JG, *et al.* Tumor-associated neutrophils stimulate T cell responses in early-stage human lung cancer. J Clin Invest 2014; 124(12): 5466-80.
[http://dx.doi.org/10.1172/JCI77053] [PMID: 25384214]

[97]   Bruno A, Ferlazzo G, Albini A, Noonan DM. A think tank of TINK/TANKs: tumor-infiltrating/tumo--associated natural killer cells in tumor progression and angiogenesis. J Natl Cancer Inst 2014; 106(8): dju200.
[http://dx.doi.org/10.1093/jnci/dju200] [PMID: 25178695]

[98]   Chen D, Jiao Y, Torquato S. A cellular automaton model for tumor dormancy: emergence of a proliferative switch. PLoS One 2014; 9(10): e109934.
[http://dx.doi.org/10.1371/journal.pone.0109934] [PMID: 25329892]

[99]   Aguirre-Ghiso JA, Bragado P, Sosa MS. Metastasis awakening: targeting dormant cancer. Nat Med 2013; 19(3): 276-7. [Metastasis awakening: targeting dormant cancer.].
[http://dx.doi.org/10.1038/nm.3120] [PMID: 23467238]

[100] Lin WC, Rajbhandari N, Liu C, *et al.* Dormant cancer cells contribute to residual disease in a model of reversible pancreatic cancer. Cancer Res 2013; 73(6): 1821-30.
[http://dx.doi.org/10.1158/0008-5472.CAN-12-2067] [PMID: 23467612]

[101] El Touny LH, Vieira A, Mendoza A, Khanna C, Hoenerhoff MJ, Green JE. Combined SFK/MEK

inhibition prevents metastatic outgrowth of dormant tumor cells. J Clin Invest 2014; 124(1): 156-68.
[http://dx.doi.org/10.1172/JCI70259] [PMID: 24316974]

[102]   Endo H, Okuyama H, Ohue M, Inoue M. Dormancy of cancer cells with suppression of AKT activity contributes to survival in chronic hypoxia. PLoS One 2014; 9(6): e98858.
[http://dx.doi.org/10.1371/journal.pone.0098858] [PMID: 24905002]

[103]   Ilie M, Hofman V, Long-Mira E, *et al.* "Sentinel" circulating tumor cells allow early diagnosis of lung cancer in patients with chronic obstructive pulmonary disease. PLoS One 2014; 9(10): e111597.
[http://dx.doi.org/10.1371/journal.pone.0111597] [PMID: 25360587]

[104]   Madic J, Kiialainen A, Bidard FC, *et al.* Circulating tumor DNA and circulating tumor cells in metastatic triple negative breast cancer patients. Int J Cancer 2015; 136(9): 2158-65.
[http://dx.doi.org/10.1002/ijc.29265] [PMID: 25307450]

[105]   Ignatiadis M, Dawson SJ. Circulating tumor cells and circulating tumor DNA for precision medicine: dream or reality? Ann Oncol 2014; 25(12): 2304-13.
[http://dx.doi.org/10.1093/annonc/mdu480] [PMID: 25336116]

[106]   Ting DT, Wittner BS, Ligorio M, *et al.* Single-cell RNA sequencing identifies extracellular matrix gene expression by pancreatic circulating tumor cells. Cell Reports 2014; 8(6): 1905-18.
[http://dx.doi.org/10.1016/j.celrep.2014.08.029] [PMID: 25242334]

[107]   Aceto N, Bardia A, Miyamoto DT, *et al.* Circulating tumor cell clusters are oligoclonal precursors of breast cancer metastasis. Cell 2014; 158(5): 1110-22.
[http://dx.doi.org/10.1016/j.cell.2014.07.013] [PMID: 25171411]

[108]   Joosse SA, Gorges TM, Pantel K. Biology, detection, and clinical implications of circulating tumor cells. EMBO Mol Med 2015; 7(1): 1-11.
[http://dx.doi.org/10.15252/emmm.201303698] [PMID: 25398926]

[109]   Deng Y, Zhang Y, Sun S, *et al.* An integrated microfluidic chip system for single-cell secretion profiling of rare circulating tumor cells. Sci Rep 2014; 4: 7499.
[http://dx.doi.org/10.1038/srep07499] [PMID: 25511131]

[110]   Hoffmann A, Levchenko A, Scott ML, Baltimore D. The IkappaB-NF-kappaB signaling module: temporal control and selective gene activation. Science 2002; 298(5596): 1241-5.
[http://dx.doi.org/10.1126/science.1071914] [PMID: 12424381]

[111]   Krishna S, Jensen MH, Sneppen K. Minimal model of spiky oscillations in NF-kappaB signaling. Proc Natl Acad Sci USA 2006; 103(29): 10840-5.
[http://dx.doi.org/10.1073/pnas.0604085103] [PMID: 16829571]

[112]   Varadhachary GR, Raber MN. Cancer of unknown primary site. N Engl J Med 2014; 371(8): 757-65.
[http://dx.doi.org/10.1056/NEJMra1303917] [PMID: 25140961]

[113]   Moller AK, Loft A, Berthelsen AK, *et al.* 18F-FDG PET/CT as a diagnostic tool in patients with extracervical carcinoma of unknown primary site: a literature review. Oncologist 2011; 16(4): 445-51.
[http://dx.doi.org/10.1634/theoncologist.2010-0189] [PMID: 21427201]

CHAPTER 5

Cancer Stem Cell and Clinical Cancer Metastasis in Surgical Oncology

Shoji Nakamori[1,*] and **Koji Morimoto**[1,2]

[1] *Department of Hepato-Biliary-Pancreatic Surgery, Osaka National Hospital, Osaka, Japan*

[2] *Osaka Women's Junior College, Osaka, Japan*

Abstract: The cancer stem cell (CSC) theory has emerged as an attractive hypothesis for tumor development and progression including metastasis. The theory suggests that tumors consist of subsets of cells with functional heterogeneity in which one small subset has the characteristics of stem cells. These stem cells have the capacity of both self-renewal and heterogeneous differentiation into cancer cells that comprise the tumor. They can also play an important role in invasion, metastasis and, finally, recurrence. Based on the pathgenesis of the cancer metastasis, the recurrences after curative surgery probably develop from the proliferation of occult micro-metastases already established at the time of surgery. The attractive ideas about CSCs hypothesis in metastasis can partially explain the concept of minimal residual disease like occult micro-metastases after curative resections. CSC hypothesis in clinical metastasis is now giving a deep impact on surgical oncology. Efforts to develop diagnostic and therapeutic approach with the successful results from CSC studies would lead to impressive improvement for cancer patients in surgery.

Keywords: Adjuvant chemotherapy, Biomarker, Cancer, Cancer stem cell (CSC), Circulating tumor cells (CTC), Disseminating tumor cells (DTC), Epithelial-mesencymal transition (EMT), Mesenchymal-epithelial transition (MET), Metastasis, Micro-metastases, Prognosis, Recurrence, R0 resection, Surgery, Surgical oncology, Target therapy.

[*] **Corresponding author Shoji Nakamori:** Department of Hepatobiliary-Pancreatic Surgery, Osaka National Hospital, 2-1-14, Hoenzaka, Chuo-ku, Osaka, 540-0006, Japan; Tel: +81-6-6942-1331; Fax: +81-6-6943-6467; Email: nakamori@onh.go.jp.

Takanori Kawaguchi (Ed.)

INTRODUCTION

Cancer metastasis consists of a multistage process during which cancer cells spread from the primary to distant organs [1]. At first, cancer cells detach from the extracellular matrix and invade the surrounding tissue. Cancer cells migrate toward a vascular blood supply by localized proteolysis at the tumor cell-basement membrane interface and then, penetrate thin-walled vessels to gain access to the systemic circulation (intravasation). Cancer cells circulate as individual cells or clusters with some blood components like platelets and arrest in the distant microvascular beds by passive or active mechanisms. Cancer cells migrate into arrested remote organ through the endothelial cells (extravasation) by multiple mechanisms. Adherent cancer cells may migrate across intracellular junctions between adjacent endothelial cells (paracellular route) or they may penetrate through the body of a single endothelial cell (transcellular route). After gaining access to the underlying tissue of arrested remote organ, cancer cells establish reciprocal signaling networks with surrounding stromal cells to promote their growth including neo-vascularization and finally establish metastatic focus. To survive through the multistage process, cancer cells should possess the ability to escape from physical pressures in the vascular stream, anoikis, apoptosis, and the host's immunologic defenses. Although the rate of cancer cell release in cancer patients is unknown, metastasis is regarded as a highly inefficient process in that less than 0.01% of circulating cancer cells eventually succeeds in forming secondary tumor growth by experimental model [2]. This is a result of the elimination of circulating tumor cells that fail to complete all steps in the metastatic process. The metastatic process is realized to be inefficient [3]. Therefore, it has been debatable whether a few cancer cells with fortunate survival and growth can develop the metastasis or whether a unique subpopulation of cancer cells with selective properties for growth and survival can develop the metastasis [4]. However, a lot of findings based on animal models and clinical studies suggest that human tumors are biologically heterogeneous [5] and that the process of clinical metastasis is selective [6].

Recently, the cancer stem cell (CSC) theory has emerged as an attractive hypothesis for tumor development and progression including metastasis [7, 8]. The theory suggests that tumors consist of subsets of cells with functional heterogeneity in which one small subset has the characteristics of stem cells. These stem cells have the capacity of both self-renewal and heterogeneous differentiation into cancer cells that comprise the tumor [7]. They can also play an important role in invasion, metastasis and, finally, recurrence. Based on the recent findings, CSCs can induce cancer metastasis through multiple pathways and participate in angiogenesis directly and indirectly [9 - 11]. Furthermore, the migrating cancer stem cell concept [12] proposed that CSCs *in situ* can transform to migrating cancer stem cells by epithelial-mesencymal transition (EMT). Then, they disseminate and form metastatic foci. Indeed, cells possessing both the stem and tumorigenic phenotypes of CSCs were derived from human mammary epithelial cells [13].

In this review, impact of CSCs in clinical metastasis is overviewed from surgical oncologist's aspects.

CLINICAL SIGNIFICANCE OF METASTASIS IN SURGERY

Despite the recent advances in diagnostic techniques for early detection of cancer and the progress in therapeutic procedures including surgical resection, chemotherapy, and radiation therapy, prognosis of the patients with cancers is still unsatisfactory. Major problems for the cancer treatment are not the primary tumors but the formation of metastases [14]. Recurrence is the most critical situation in the treatment of cancer patients after curative surgery. Almost all of cancer recurrences are due to metastasis on the distant organs or regional lymph nodes if surgical resection is undergone in curative intent. Clinically, patients with distant metastasis are hardly appropriate to surgical resection which possibly offers the patients with solid cancer an opportunity to live longer and cure. Even though patients underwent curative resection (surgical macroscopically zero residual: R0) resections at the surgery, a significant number of the patients have recurrence with developing systemic metastasis at distant organ within a few years after surgery. Main reason of cancer death remains to be recurrence due to the metastasis. Based on the pathogenesis of the cancer metastasis, these recurrences probably develop from the proliferation of occult micro-metastases already established at the time of surgery [15, 16]. Clinical metastasis, however, detected after surgery varies from patient to patient. Multiple liver metastases sometimes develop within a few weeks after curative resection for pancreatic cancer (Fig. **1**), while no apparent distant metastasis has been detected over 7 years after diagnosis in spite of growth of primary tumor even in patient with pancreatic cancer of dismal prognosis (Fig. **2**). Although the attractive ideas about CSCs hypothesis in metastasis can partially explain the concept of minimal residual disease like occult micro-metastases after curative resections, there can be a possibility that clinical metastasis originated from none CSCs (Fig. **3**).

(a) **(b)**

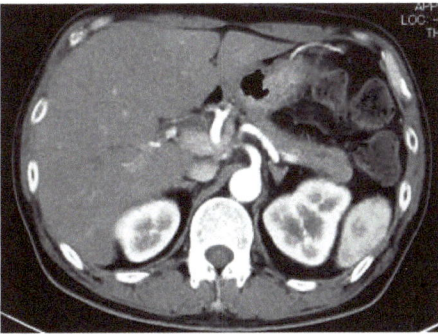 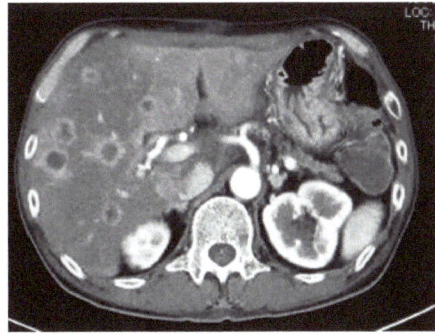

Fig. (1). Computed tomography before surgery (**a**) and 6 weeks after R0 pancreaticoduodenectomy for pancreas head cancer (**b**). Multiple liver metastases appeared within 6 weeks after surgery.

(a) **(b)**

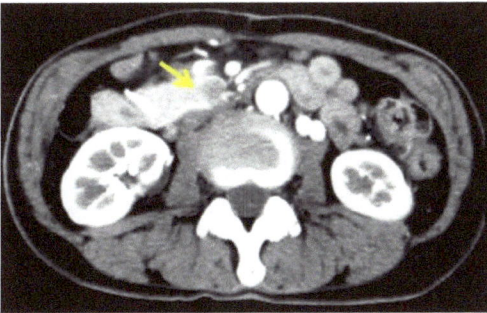 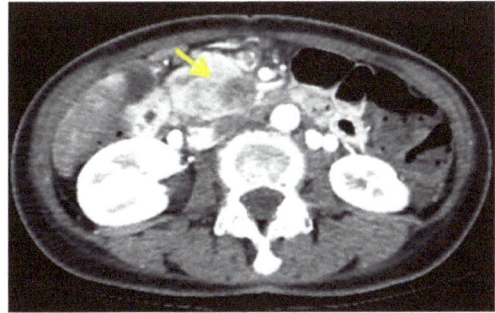

Fig. (2). Computed tomography on pancreatic cancer (arrow) diagnosed (**a**) and on 7 years after diagnosis without treatment (**b**). No apparent metastases have been revealed during 7 years.

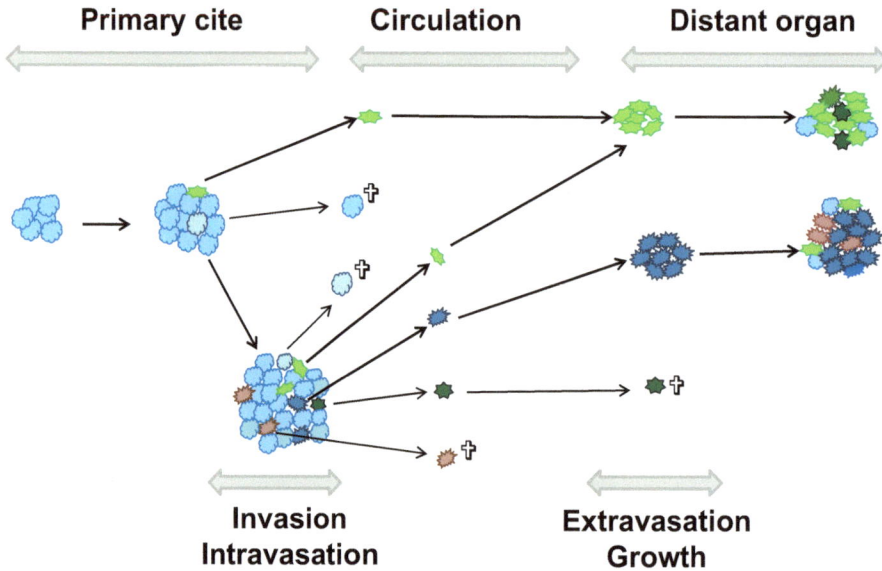

Fig. (3). Tumor development and metastasis. Subpopulations including both cancer stem cells and non-cancer stem cells in primary tumor may have metastatic potential. Cancer cells that released from primary site hardly survive in circulation or in arrested organs (✟). Both the cells within the primary tumor and metastatic lesions can continue to diversify as the lesions grow.

BIOMARKERS OF CSC

It is widely acceptable that metastasis arises from a tumor cell subpopulation of higher metastatic potential within the primary tumor [15]. Highly metastatic tumor cells may exhibit a variety of biochemical features that differ from those of their less metastatic counterparts. These cells are thought to arise within the primary tumors and become predominant [16]. Therefore, the identification of specific indicators of metastatic potential at the time of diagnosis or surgery for primary

tumors has been focused to allow a better prognostic evaluation of the patient, and hence a better therapeutic approach [17]. Thus, unique repertories of surface biomarker expressed in CSCs should be investigated not only for their reliable isolation from non-tumorigenic cells in bench, but also for clinical applications in bed side.

The ability to form tumors in immunodeficient mice by xenograft transplantation and tumorsphere formation in non-adherence 3D cultures were utilized to confirm the CSCs in bench. As few as 100 isolated transplanted CSCs can successfully develop tumor in xenograft models [18 - 20]. CSCs were initially identified in acute myeloid leukemia as $CD34^+/CD38^-$ subpopulation [21]. Appropriate cell surface markers used for identification and isolation of CSCs varied on the organ to organ. Since the first pioneering studies in acute myeloid leukemia, such extensive efforts have been undertaken to identify biomarkers able to recognize CSCs among highly abundant differentiated cancer cells. Biomarkers for CSCs have been recognized in a wide variety of human cancers (Table **1**).

Table 1. Biomarkers for detection of cancer stem cells.

Tumor Type	Cell Surface Biomarker and Phenotype	Reference
Acute myeloid leukemia	$CD34^+/CD38^-$, CD34+/CD38+, CD25, CD33, CD52, CD96, CD123	[21 - 27]
Acute lymphoid leukemia	$CD34^+/CD19^-$, $CD34^+/CD38^-/CD19^+$, $CD34^+/CD19^+$	[28 - 30]
Chronic lymphoid leukemia	$CD34^+/CD19^+$	[31]
Myeloma	$CD20^+/CD27^+/CD138^-$	[32]
Gliobrastoma	$CD133^+$, $CD15^+/CD133^+$, $CD133^+/SSEA-1^+$	[33 - 35]
Head and neck cancer	$CD44^+/$ $CK5/14^+/BMI-1^+$	[36, 37]
Breast Cancer	$CD44^+/$ $CD24^-/ESA^+$, $CD44^+/CD24^{low}/lin^-/ALDH1^+$, $CD44^+/CD24^{low/-}$, $CD326^+/CD45^-/CD44^+/CD24^-$, $CD44^+/CD49f^-/CD133^+$, MET^+	[18, 19, 38 - 42]
Small cell lung cancer	$CD133^+$	[43]
Non-small cell lung cancer	$Sca^+/CD45^-/PECAM^-/CD34^+$, $CD133^+$	[44, 45]
Gastric cancer	$CD133^+/CD44^+$, $CD326^+/CD44^+$, $CD49f^-$	[46 - 48]
Liver cancer	$CD133^+$, $EpCAM^+/AFP^+$, $CD44^+/CD90^+$	[49 - 51]
Pancreatic cancer	$CD44^+/CD24^+/CD326^+$, $CD133^+/CXCR4^+$	[52, 53]
Colorectal cancer	$CD133^+$, $CD326^+/CD44^+/$ $CD166^+$, $CD44^+/CD49^{f+}/CD133^+$	[20, 54, 55]
Prostate cancer	$CD44^+/CD49^f/CD326^+$, $CD44^+/CD24^-$, $CD44^+/CD133^+$	[56 - 58]
Bladder cancer	$EMA^-/CD44v6^+$	[59]
Ovarian cancer	$CD44^+/CD49^f/CD326^+$, $CD44^+/CD117^+$, $CD133^+$	[60 - 62]
Osteosarcoma	$CD117^+/STRO-1^+$, $CD133^+$, $CD271^+$	[63 - 65]
Ewing's sarcoma	$CD133^+$	[66]
Melanoma	CD271+, ABCB5+, EPOR+	[67 - 69]

CSC AND PROGNOSIS

CSCs have three main characteristics [7, 8, 70 - 73]. First, they have the similarities in the mechanisms that regulate self-renewal and differentiation of normal stem cells and cancer cells. Second, they have the capacity to maintain the stem cell pool, and third, sustain the heterogeneous growth of cancer lesions and generate all the cell types observed not only in the primary tumor but also in metastatic tumors.

In a complex process of metastatic cascade, epithelial-mesencymal transition (EMT) is accepted as an essential procedure in early step of metastasis of release from primary tumor [74, 75]. Mesenchymal-epithelial transition (MET) is a reverse process of EMT and called as re-differentiation process [75]. MET is also accepted as an essential procedure in late step of metastasis of colonization and formation of micrometastasis. ENT-MET transition processes are accepted as a driving force of metastasis [76, 77]. CSCs have linked to ENT-MET transition in the cell plasticity, which is one of the main CSCs properties, and thus, are recognized to play an important role in metastasis and finally, prognosis of their patients. Furthermore, a majority proportion of disseminating tumor cells (DTC) detected in bone marrow of breast cancer patients share a cancer stem cell marker phenotype [78]. A large proportion of circulating tumor cells (CTC) isolated from primary or metastatic breast cancer patients share stem cell phenotype and EMT characteristics [79].

Based on the above concept including EMT, MET, DTCs, and CTCs [80], CSCs are thought to play a significant role in development of clinical metastasis and can be detected in surgical samples due to biological heterogeneity of cancer cells in primary tumor. To date, several clinicopathologic characteristics based on morphologic features, *i.e.*; histologic type of the lesion, the mode of cancer invasion, the presence of lymph-node metastasis and, most importantly, pathologic stage based on above factors have been considered to be important indicators of prognosis in assessing the potential malignancy of almost all of cancer to evaluate the risk of recurrence [81 - 85]. However, the patients' prognosis within a single stage is not the same, particularly within the earlier stages of the disease. Therefore, since the clinicopathologic stratification is based on the above morphologic characterization, additional factors implicated in the biologic function affecting tumor progression and metastasis should be sought to identify subgroups among patients within the same stage who are most at risk for tumor recurrence and death [86, 87]. Recently, detection of CSCs is recognized as an indicator of patients' prognosis. Indeed, CSCs detected by ALDH1 (Aldehyde dehydrogenase 1) expression are observed in surgically resected breast cancer tumors (Fig. **4**) and patients with ALDH1 strong positive tumors have worse relapse free survival [40] (Fig. **5**). Resent aggressive studies also demonstrated that the presence of CSCs in human tumor specimen resected at surgery has correlated with poor prognosis across many organs (Table **2**).

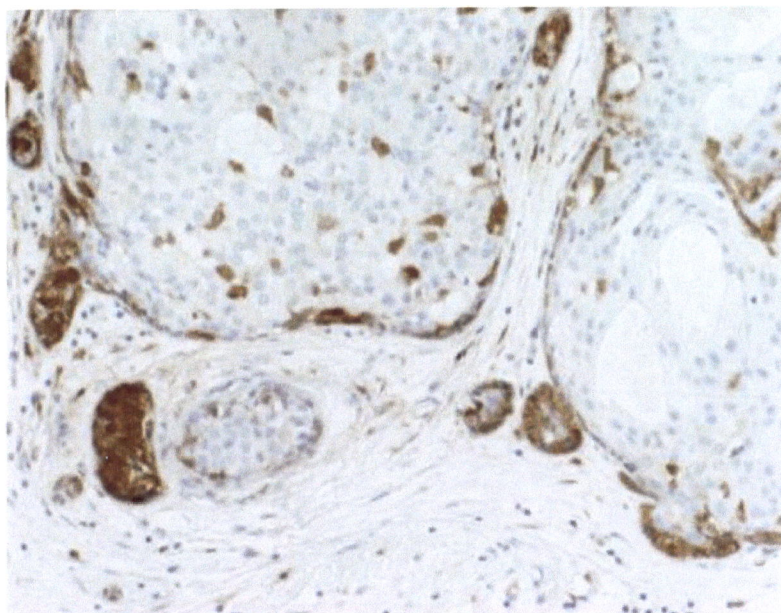

Fig. (4). Immunohistochemical detection of ALDH1 (Aldehyde dehydrogenase 1) expression in surgically resected breast cancer tissue.

Table 2. Correlation of worse patient's prognosis and biomarker expression related to CSCs.

Tumor Type	Biomarker Used	Reference
Head and neck cancer	Bmi-1(tongue), Oct4 (hypopharyngeal), CD98(HPV+ oropharyngeal)	[88 - 90]
Breast Cancer	ALDH1$^+$, CD44$^+$, CD133$^+$, Bmi-1, CD44$^+$/CD24$^-$	[40, 91 - 95]
Lung cancer	CD133$^+$, ALDH1$^+$	[96 - 98]

(Table 2) contd.....

Tumor Type	Biomarker Used	Reference
Gastric cancer	CD133$^+$, CD44$^+$, CD44$^+$/ CD326$^-$	[99 - 101]
Liver cancer	EpCAM$^+$/AFP$^+$, CD133$^+$, HIWI, CD90$^+$	[102 - 105]
Pancreatic cancer	ALDH1$^-$, CD44$^+$/CD24$^+$, CD44$^+$/CD133$^+$	[106 - 108]
Colorectal cancer	CD133+, ALDH1$^+$	[109, 110]
Prostate cancer	CD44$^+$/CD24$^-$, ALDH1$^+$, OCT4$^+$, CD44$^+$/CD133$^+$	[57, 111, 112]
Bladder cancer	ALDH1$^+$	[113]
Ovarian cancer	CD133$^+$, ALDH1+, CD44$^+$/CD24$^-$	[114 - 116]
Soft tissue sarcoma	LGR5$^+$/GPR49$^+$	[117]

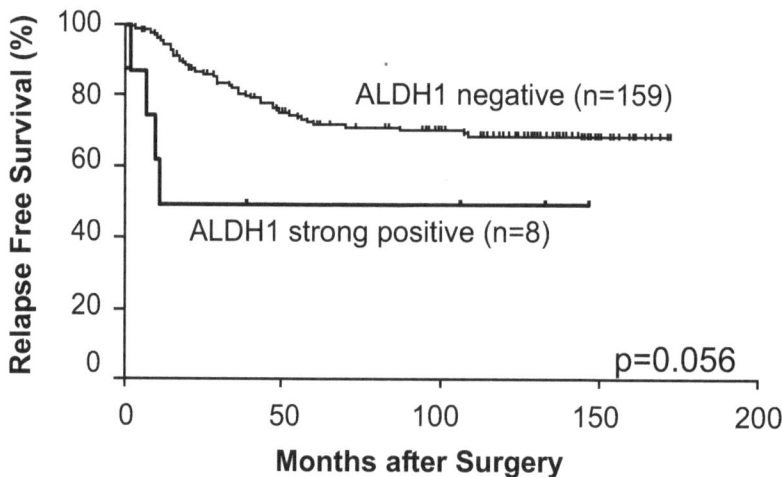

Fig. (5). Relapse free survival curves according to ALDH1 expression for 167 patients who underwent curative resection for breast cancer. One hundred fifty nine patients had ALDH1 negative tumors (faint line) and 8 patients had strong positive tumors (solid line). The difference between the two curves tended to be significant (p=0.056, log rank test).

CSC AND THERAPEUTIC APPLICATION IN SURGERY

Although neo-adjuvant and post-operative adjuvant chemotherapy and radiation are widely applied to reduce the relapse and metastasis rate after surgery, mortality rate for cancers in a variety of organs still remains to be unfavorable. This disappoint results can be partially explained with some properties of CSCs [4, 80, 118]. Firstly, CSCs with metastasizing potential is acquired in the very early stage of the cancer life. These CSCs have already seeded at metastatic sites when cancer was clinically diagnosed and treated even at early stage. Almost all of them are gradually growing up at the seeded sites and be apparent after surgery, though the growing speed of them varies from cancer cell to cancer cell or from organ to organ. They sometimes can remain in a dormant status and give rise to disease after long period of post-R0 cancer free. Secondly, CSCs possess unique protection mechanisms including expression of ABC transporter proteins, enhanced DNA repair mechanisms and resistant to DNA damage, and expression of anti-apoptoic proteins, which reduce sensitivity against therapeutic agents and make CSCs resistant to chemo and radiation therapy [119 - 121]. Although post-operative adjuvant chemotherapy is widely accepted to target occult micro-metastases after R0 resection, it cannot always prevent the recurrence not only because of its ineffectiveness to cancer cells but also chemoresistance of CSCs in occult micro-metastases. Actually, cancer cells with the characteristics of CSCs are detected from the primary and metastatic sites after chemotherapy (Fig. **6**). An increasing number of studies show that CSCs are involved in resistance to chemotherapy and radiotherapy in variety of organs including breast, lung, colon, ovary, and pancreas [122 - 126]. Taken together, CSCs are thought to play an important role in chemo and radiation resistance and can make a pre- or post-adjuvant treatment after surgery vain. Therefore, clinical strategies against specifically targeting CSCs are reasonable and have been vigorously developed since CSCs theory is established.

To date, there are four main strategies for CSC-target therapies in cancer treatment which include increasing sensitization of CSCs to conventional chemotherapeutic agents, promoting CSC differentiation, targeting and blocking relevant CSC signaling pathways, and destroying CSC niches [121]. Because CSCs insensitive to conventional chemotherapy like normal stem cells make them difficult to eliminate completely, increasing sensitivity of CSCs to conventional therapy is crucial to improve chemotherapeutic effects. Recent aggressive efforts with CSCs demonstrated that signaling pathways, such as Wnt, Notch, and Hedgehog are essential for regulation of EMT- change, differentiation and self-renewal of CSCs in several cancers. Although development of agents that target these signaling pathways will be complicated due to these cross-talk and influence on non-CSCs cells, several agents targeting signal pathways in CSCs have been developed. These agents combined with/without conventional chemotherapeutic drugs are promising in clinical trials for inoperable cancers with gross primary tumors with/without multiple metastases (Table **3**), though CSCs target therapy can be theoretically the most suitable for adjuvant therapy for patients with R0 resection. Recently, these therapies were applied for adjuvant treatment in breast cancer and resulted were controversial [140, 141].

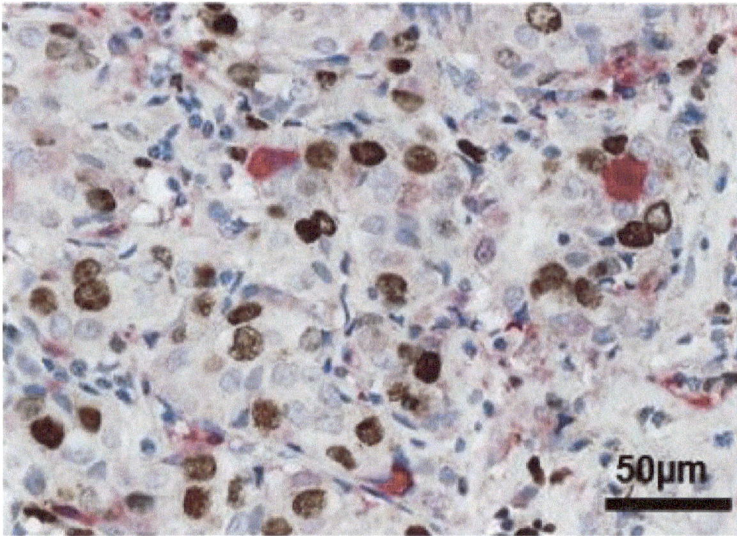

Fig. (6). Double immunohistochemical detection of ALDH1 (red) and Ki-67(brown) in surgically resected breast cancer tumor after neo-adjuvant chemotherapy. After chemotherapy, the resistant cancer stem cells present in the tissue are positive for ALDH1 and negative for Ki-67. Non cancer stem cells positive for Ki-67 are also observed, which survived after the conventional chemotherapy.

Table 3. Target molecules and phenotype related to CSCs in solid tumors.

Target type	Target molecule	Tumor type	Drug	Reference
Signaling pathways	Hedgehog	Skin cancer	Vismodegib	[127]
	BRAF	Melanoma	Vemurafenib	[128]
	mTOR	Glioblastoma	Temisirolimus	[129]
		Renal cancer	Temisirolimus	[130]
Cytokine receptors	EGFR	Pancreatic cancer	Erlotinib	[131]
	ERBB2	Breast cancer	Lapatinib	[132]
	KIT, PDGER	GIST	Imatinib	[133]

(Table 3) contd.....

Target type	Target molecule	Tumor type	Drug	Reference
Surface antigen	EGFR	Colorectal cancer	Cetuximab	[134, 135]
	HER2	Breast cancer	Trastuzumab	[136]
	EGFR/HER1,HER3, HER4		Pertuzumab	[137]
	HER2	Gastric cancer	Trastzumab	[138]
		Ovarian cancer	Trastzumab	[139]

Other strategy is to destroy CSC-dependent stem cell niches, in which signaling pathways initiate and facilitate tumor formation and components in the micro-environment protect CSCs against chemotherapy. Therefore, extracellular matrix and soluble factors for angiogenesis and lymphangiogenesis in CSC niches may be potent target therapy [121, 142]. Inhibitor of vascular endothelial growth factor receptor (VEGFR) with chemotherapeutic agents has already been used in clinic [143 - 145] but is still undergoing for adjuvant therapy after R0 resection [146 - 150].

CONCLUSION

Although the cancer stem cell theory is provocative to investigate and understand clinical cancer metastasis, it has not been recognized enough to develop and utilize the new strategies to treat cancer patients in the field of surgical oncology. It still remains obscure that CSCs resulted in all of the recurrence due to metastasis after R0 resection. We should keep not only to develop the technology for the detection of cancer in their early stages but also to improve the surgical techniques for R0 resection. These efforts combined with the successful results from CSC studies could bring impressive improvement for cancer patients.

CONFLICT OF INTEREST

The authors confirm that they have no conflict of interest to declare for this publication.

ACKNOWLEDGEMENTS

This work was supported in part by the National Cancer Center Research and Development Funds and the Grant-in-Aid for Clinical Cancer Research from the

Ministry of Health, Labour and Welfare of Japan.

REFERENCES

[1]   Nguyen DX, Bos PD, Massagué J. Metastasis: from dissemination to organ-specific colonization. Nat Rev Cancer 2009; 9(4): 274-84.
[PMID: 19308067]

[2]   Fidler IJ. Metastasis: quantitative analysis of distribution and fate of tumor emboli labeled with 125 I-5-iodo-2′-deoxyuridine. J Natl Cancer Inst 1970; 45(4): 773-82.
[PMID: 5513503]

[3]   Weiss L. Metastatic inefficiency: cause and consequences. Cancer Rev 1986; 3: 1-24.

[4]   Talmadge JE, Fidler IJ. AACR centennial series: the biology of cancer metastasis: historical perspective. Cancer Res 2010; 70(14): 5649-69.
[PMID: 20610625]

[5]   Chiang AC, Massagué J. Molecular basis of metastasis. N Engl J Med 2008; 359(26): 2814-23.
[PMID: 19109576]

[6]   Kuukasjärvi T, Karhu R, Tanner M, *et al.* Genetic heterogeneity and clonal evolution underlying development of asynchronous metastasis in human breast cancer. Cancer Res 1997; 57(8): 1597-604.
[PMID: 9108466]

[7]   Reya T, Morrison SJ, Clarke MF, Weissman IL. Stem cells, cancer, and cancer stem cells. Nature 2001; 414(6859): 105-11.
[PMID: 11689955]

[8]   Li F, Tiede B, Massagué J, Kang Y. Beyond tumorigenesis: cancer stem cells in metastasis. Cell Res 2007; 17(1): 3-14.
[PMID: 17179981]

[9]   Clarke MF, Dick JE, Dirks PB, *et al.* Cancer stem cells--perspectives on current status and future directions: AACR Workshop on cancer stem cells. Cancer Res 2006; 66(19): 9339-44.
[PMID: 16990346]

[10]   Bjerkvig R, Johansson M, Miletic H, Niclou SP. Cancer stem cells and angiogenesis. Semin Cancer Biol 2009; 19(5): 279-84.
[PMID: 19818406]

[11]   Yao XH, Ping YF, Bian XW. Contribution of cancer stem cells to tumor vasculogenic mimicry. Protein Cell 2011; 2(4): 266-72.
[PMID: 21533771]

[12]   Brabletz T, Jung A, Spaderna S, Hlubek F, Kirchner T. Opinion: migrating cancer stem cells - an integrated concept of malignant tumour progression. Nat Rev Cancer 2005; 5(9): 744-9.
[PMID: 16148886]

[13]   Gudjonsson T, Villadsen R, Nielsen HL, Rønnov-Jessen L, Bissell MJ, Petersen OW. Isolation, immortalization, and characterization of a human breast epithelial cell line with stem cell properties. Genes Dev 2002; 16(6): 693-706.
[PMID: 11914275]

[14] Hanahan D, Weinberg RA. Hallmarks of cancer: the next generation. Cell 2011; 144(5): 646-74.
[PMID: 21376230]

[15] Fidler IJ, Kripke ML. Metastasis results from preexisting variant cells within a malignant tumor. Science 1977; 197(4306): 893-5.
[PMID: 887927]

[16] Nicolson GL. Generation of phenotypic diversity and progression in metastatic tumor cells. Cancer Metastasis Rev 1984; 3(1): 25-42.
[PMID: 6370418]

[17] Hellman S, Weichselbaum RR. Oligometastases. J Clin Oncol 1995; 13(1): 8-10.
[PMID: 7799047]

[18] Al-Hajj M, Wicha MS, Benito-Hernandez A, Morrison SJ, Clarke MF. Prospective identification of tumorigenic breast cancer cells. Proc Natl Acad Sci USA 2003; 100(7): 3983-8.
[PMID: 12629218]

[19] Jordan CT, Guzman ML, Noble M. Cancer stem cells. N Engl J Med 2006; 355(12): 1253-61.
[PMID: 16990388]

[20] Ricci-Vitiani L, Lombardi DG, Pilozzi E, et al. Identification and expansion of human colon-cance--initiating cells. Nature 2007; 445(7123): 111-5.
[PMID: 17122771]

[21] Bonnet D, Dick JE. Human acute myeloid leukemia is organized as a hierarchy that originates from a primitive hematopoietic cell. Nat Med 1997; 3(7): 730-7.
[PMID: 9212098]

[22] Taussig DC, Miraki-Moud F, Anjos-Afonso F, et al. Anti-CD38 antibody-mediated clearance of human repopulating cells masks the heterogeneity of leukemia-initiating cells. Blood 2008; 112(3): 568-75.
[PMID: 18523148]

[23] Saito Y, Kitamura H, Hijikata A, et al. Identification of therapeutic targets for quiescent, chemotherapy-resistant human leukemia stem cells. Sci Transl Med 2010; 2(17): 17ra9.
[PMID: 20371479]

[24] Taussig DC, Pearce DJ, Simpson C, et al. Hematopoietic stem cells express multiple myeloid markers: implications for the origin and targeted therapy of acute myeloid leukemia. Blood 2005; 106(13): 4086-92.
[PMID: 16131573]

[25] Blatt K, Herrmann H, Hoermann G, et al. Identification of campath-1 (CD52) as novel drug target in neoplastic stem cells in 5q-patients with MDS and AML. Clin Cancer Res 2014; 20(13): 3589-602.
[PMID: 24799522]

[26] Hosen N, Park CY, Tatsumi N, et al. CD96 is a leukemic stem cell-specific marker in human acute myeloid leukemia. Proc Natl Acad Sci USA 2007; 104(26): 11008-13.
[PMID: 17576927]

[27] Jordan CT, Upchurch D, Szilvassy SJ, et al. The interleukin-3 receptor alpha chain is a unique marker for human acute myelogenous leukemia stem cells. Leukemia 2000; 14(10): 1777-84.

[PMID: 11021753]

[28]   Cox CV, Evely RS, Oakhill A, Pamphilon DH, Goulden NJ, Blair A. Characterization of acute lymphoblastic leukemia progenitor cells. Blood 2004; 104(9): 2919-25.
[PMID: 15242869]

[29]   Cobaleda C, Gutiérrez-Cianca N, Pérez-Losada J, *et al.* A primitive hematopoietic cell is the target for the leukemic transformation in human philadelphia-positive acute lymphoblastic leukemia. Blood 2000; 95(3): 1007-13.
[PMID: 10648416]

[30]   Kong Y, Yoshida S, Saito Y, *et al.* CD34+CD38+CD19+ as well as CD34+CD38-CD19+ cells are leukemia-initiating cells with self-renewal capacity in human B-precursor ALL. Leukemia 2008; 22(6): 1207-13.
[PMID: 18418410]

[31]   Rossi FM, Zucchetto A, Tissino E, *et al.* CD49d expression identifies a chronic-lymphocytic leukemia subset with high levels of mobilized circulating CD34(+) hemopoietic progenitors cells. Leukemia 2014; 28(3): 705-8.
[PMID: 24202404]

[32]   Matsui W, Wang Q, Barber JP, *et al.* Clonogenic multiple myeloma progenitors, stem cell properties, and drug resistance. Cancer Res 2008; 68(1): 190-7.
[PMID: 18172311]

[33]   Singh SK, Clarke ID, Terasaki M, *et al.* Identification of a cancer stem cell in human brain tumors. Cancer Res 2003; 63(18): 5821-8.
[PMID: 14522905]

[34]   Kahlert UD, Bender NO, Maciaczyk D, *et al.* CD133/CD15 defines distinct cell subpopulations with differential *in vitro* clonogenic activity and stem cell-related gene expression profile in *in vitro* propagated glioblastoma multiforme-derived cell line with a PNET-like component. Folia Neuropathol 2012; 50(4): 357-68.
[PMID: 23319191]

[35]   Son MJ, Woolard K, Nam DH, Lee J, Fine HA. SSEA-1 is an enrichment marker for tumor-initiating cells in human glioblastoma. Cell Stem Cell 2009; 4(5): 440-52.
[PMID: 19427293]

[36]   Costea DE, Tsinkalovsky O, Vintermyr OK, Johannessen AC, Mackenzie IC. Cancer stem cells - new and potentially important targets for the therapy of oral squamous cell carcinoma. Oral Dis 2006; 12(5): 443-54.
[PMID: 16910914]

[37]   Prince ME, Sivanandan R, Kaczorowski A, *et al.* Identification of a subpopulation of cells with cancer stem cell properties in head and neck squamous cell carcinoma. Proc Natl Acad Sci USA 2007; 104(3): 973-8.
[PMID: 17210912]

[38]   Bomken S, Fiser K, Heidenreich O, Vormoor J. Understanding the cancer stem cell. Br J Cancer 2010; 103(4): 439-45.
[PMID: 20664590]

[39]   Lum LG, Fok H, Sievers R, Abedi M, Quesenberry PJ, Lee RJ. Targeting of Lin-Sca+ hematopoietic stem cells with bispecific antibodies to injured myocardium. Blood Cells Mol Dis 2004; 32(1): 82-7. [PMID: 14757418]

[40]   Morimoto K, Kim SJ, Tanei T, *et al.* Stem cell marker aldehyde dehydrogenase 1-positive breast cancers are characterized by negative estrogen receptor, positive human epidermal growth factor receptor type 2, and high Ki67 expression. Cancer Sci 2009; 100(6): 1062-8. [PMID: 19385968]

[41]   Meyer MJ, Fleming JM, Lin AF, Hussnain SA, Ginsburg E, Vonderhaar BK. CD44posCD49fhiCD133/2hi defines xenograft-initiating cells in estrogen receptor-negative breast cancer. Cancer Res 2010; 70(11): 4624-33. [PMID: 20484027]

[42]   Baccelli I, Schneeweiss A, Riethdorf S, *et al.* Identification of a population of blood circulating tumor cells from breast cancer patients that initiates metastasis in a xenograft assay. Nat Biotechnol 2013; 31(6): 539-44. [PMID: 23609047]

[43]   Eramo A, Lotti F, Sette G, *et al.* Identification and expansion of the tumorigenic lung cancer stem cell population. Cell Death Differ 2008; 15(3): 504-14. [PMID: 18049477]

[44]   Tang C, Ang BT, Pervaiz S. Cancer stem cell: target for anti-cancer therapy. FASEB J 2007; 21(14): 3777-85. [PMID: 17625071]

[45]   Tirino V, Camerlingo R, Franco R, *et al.* The role of CD133 in the identification and characterisation of tumour-initiating cells in non-small-cell lung cancer. Eur J Cardiothorac Surg 2009; 36(3): 446-53. [PMID: 19464919]

[46]   Wakamatsu Y, Sakamoto N, Oo HZ, *et al.* Expression of cancer stem cell markers ALDH1, CD44 and CD133 in primary tumor and lymph node metastasis of gastric cancer. Pathol Int 2012; 62(2): 112-9. [PMID: 22243781]

[47]   Han ME, Jeon TY, Hwang SH, *et al.* Cancer spheres from gastric cancer patients provide an ideal model system for cancer stem cell research. Cell Mol Life Sci 2011; 68(21): 3589-605. [PMID: 21448722]

[48]   Fukamachi H, Seol HS, Shimada S, *et al.* CD49f(high) cells retain sphere-forming and tumor-initiating activities in human gastric tumors. PLoS One 2013; 8(8): e72438. [PMID: 24015244]

[49]   Ma S, Lee TK, Zheng BJ, Chan KW, Guan XY. CD133+ HCC cancer stem cells confer chemoresistance by preferential expression of the Akt/PKB survival pathway. Oncogene 2008; 27(12): 1749-58. [PMID: 17891174]

[50]   Yamashita T, Ji J, Budhu A, *et al.* EpCAM-positive hepatocellular carcinoma cells are tumor-initiating cells with stem/progenitor cell features. Gastroenterology 2009; 136(3): 1012-24. [PMID: 19150350]

[51]   Yang ZF, Ho DW, Ng MN, *et al.* Significance of CD90+ cancer stem cells in human liver cancer. Cancer Cell 2008; 13(2): 153-66. [PMID: 18242515]

[52]   Li C, Heidt DG, Dalerba P, *et al.* Identification of pancreatic cancer stem cells. Cancer Res 2007; 67(3): 1030-7. [PMID: 17283135]

[53]   Hermann PC, Huber SL, Herrler T, *et al.* Distinct populations of cancer stem cells determine tumor growth and metastatic activity in human pancreatic cancer. Cell Stem Cell 2007; 1(3): 313-23. [PMID: 18371365]

[54]   Dalerba P, Dylla SJ, Park IK, *et al.* Phenotypic characterization of human colorectal cancer stem cells. Proc Natl Acad Sci USA 2007; 104(24): 10158-63. [PMID: 17548814]

[55]   Haraguchi N, Ishii H, Mimori K, *et al.* CD49f-positive cell population efficiently enriches colon cancer-initiating cells. Int J Oncol 2013; 43(2): 425-30. [PMID: 23708747]

[56]   Guo C, Liu H, Zhang BH, Cadaneanu RM, Mayle AM, Garraway IP. Epcam, CD44, and CD49f distinguish sphere-forming human prostate basal cells from a subpopulation with predominant tubule initiation capability. PLoS One 2012; 7(4): e34219. [PMID: 22514625]

[57]   Hurt EM, Kawasaki BT, Klarmann GJ, Thomas SB, Farrar WL. CD44+ CD24(-) prostate cells are early cancer progenitor/stem cells that provide a model for patients with poor prognosis. Br J Cancer 2008; 98(4): 756-65. [PMID: 18268494]

[58]   Maitland NJ, Collins AT. Prostate cancer stem cells: a new target for therapy. J Clin Oncol 2008; 26(17): 2862-70. [PMID: 18539965]

[59]   Yang YM, Chang JW. Bladder cancer initiating cells (BCICs) are among EMA-CD44v6+ subset: novel methods for isolating undetermined cancer stem (initiating) cells. Cancer Invest 2008; 26(7): 725-33. [PMID: 18608209]

[60]   Meirelles K, Benedict LA, Dombkowski D, *et al.* Human ovarian cancer stem/progenitor cells are stimulated by doxorubicin but inhibited by Mullerian inhibiting substance. Proc Natl Acad Sci USA 2012; 109(7): 2358-63. [PMID: 22308459]

[61]   Chen J, Wang J, Chen D, *et al.* Evaluation of characteristics of CD44+CD117+ ovarian cancer stem cells in three dimensional basement membrane extract scaffold *versus* two dimensional monocultures. BMC Cell Biol 2013; 14: 7. [PMID: 23368632]

[62]   Curley MD, Therrien VA, Cummings CL, *et al.* CD133 expression defines a tumor initiating cell population in primary human ovarian cancer. Stem Cells 2009; 27(12): 2875-83.

[PMID: 19816957]

[63] Adhikari AS, Agarwal N, Wood BM, *et al.* CD117 and Stro-1 identify osteosarcoma tumor-initiating cells associated with metastasis and drug resistance. Cancer Res 2010; 70(11): 4602-12.
[PMID: 20460510]

[64] Tirino V, Desiderio V, Paino F, *et al.* Human primary bone sarcomas contain CD133+ cancer stem cells displaying high tumorigenicity *in vivo.* FASEB J 2011; 25(6): 2022-30.
[PMID: 21385990]

[65] Tian J, Li X, Si M, Liu T, Li J. CD271+ osteosarcoma cells display stem-like properties. PLoS One 2014; 9(6): e98549.
[PMID: 24893164]

[66] Suvà ML, Riggi N, Stehle JC, *et al.* Identification of cancer stem cells in Ewing's sarcoma. Cancer Res 2009; 69(5): 1776-81.
[PMID: 19208848]

[67] Boiko AD, Razorenova OV, van de Rijn M, *et al.* Human melanoma-initiating cells express neural crest nerve growth factor receptor CD271. Nature 2010; 466(7302): 133-7.
[PMID: 20596026]

[68] Wilson BJ, Saab KR, Ma J, *et al.* ABCB5 maintains melanoma-initiating cells through a proinflammatory cytokine signaling circuit. Cancer Res 2014; 74(15): 4196-207.
[PMID: 24934811]

[69] Mirkina I, Hadzijusufovic E, Krepler C, *et al.* Phenotyping of human melanoma cells reveals a unique composition of receptor targets and a subpopulation co-expressing ErbB4, EPO-R and NGF-R. PLoS One 2014; 9(1): e84417.
[PMID: 24489649]

[70] Reya T, Morrison SJ, Clarke MF, Weissman IL. Stem cells, cancer, and cancer stem cells. Nature 2001; 414(6859): 105-11.
[PMID: 11689955]

[71] Ailles LE, Weissman IL. Cancer stem cells in solid tumors. Curr Opin Biotechnol 2007; 18(5): 460-6.
[PMID: 18023337]

[72] Dalerba P, Cho RW, Clarke MF. Cancer stem cells: models and concepts. Annu Rev Med 2007; 58: 267-84.
[PMID: 17002552]

[73] Calabrese C, Poppleton H, Kocak M, *et al.* A perivascular niche for brain tumor stem cells. Cancer Cell 2007; 11(1): 69-82.
[PMID: 17222791]

[74] Thiery JP, Acloque H, Huang RY, Nieto MA. Epithelial-mesenchymal transitions in development and disease. Cell 2009; 139(5): 871-90.
[PMID: 19945376]

[75] Valastyan S, Weinberg RA. Tumor metastasis: molecular insights and evolving paradigms. Cell 2011; 147(2): 275-92.
[PMID: 22000009]

[76]   Brabletz T, Jung A, Reu S, *et al.* Variable beta-catenin expression in colorectal cancers indicates tumor progression driven by the tumor environment. Proc Natl Acad Sci USA 2001; 98(18): 10356-61.
[PMID: 11526241]

[77]   Tsai JH, Donaher JL, Murphy DA, Chau S, Yang J. Spatiotemporal regulation of epithelial-mesenchymal transition is essential for squamous cell carcinoma metastasis. Cancer Cell 2012; 22(6): 725-36.
[PMID: 23201165]

[78]   Balic M, Lin H, Young L, *et al.* Most early disseminated cancer cells detected in bone marrow of breast cancer patients have a putative breast cancer stem cell phenotype. Clin Cancer Res 2006; 12(19): 5615-21.
[PMID: 17020963]

[79]   Maheswaran S, Haber DA. Circulating tumor cells: a window into cancer biology and metastasis. Curr Opin Genet Dev 2010; 20(1): 96-9.
[PMID: 20071161]

[80]   Liao W-T, Ye Y-P, Deng Y-J, Bian X-W, Ding Y-Q. Metastatic cancer stem cells: from the concept to therapeutics. Am J Stem Cells 2014; 3(2): 46-62.
[PMID: 25232505]

[81]   Sobin LH, Wittekind Ch. TNM classification of malignant tumours. 7th ed., New York: Wiley-Liss 2010.

[82]   Roder JD, Böttcher K, Siewert JR, Busch R, Hermanek P, Meyer HJ. Prognostic factors in gastric carcinoma. Results of the German Gastric Carcinoma Study 1992. Cancer 1993; 72(7): 2089-97.
[PMID: 8374867]

[83]   Beahrs OH. Staging of cancer of the colon and rectum. Cancer 1992; 70(5) (Suppl.): 1393-6.
[PMID: 1511390]

[84]   Ryan DP, Hong TS, Bardeesy N. Pancreatic adenocarcinoma. N Engl J Med 2014; 371(11): 1039-49.
[PMID: 25207767]

[85]   Duseja A. Staging of hepatocellular carcinoma. J Clin Exp Hepatol 2014; 4 (Suppl. 3): S74-9.
[PMID: 25755615]

[86]   Nakamori S, Kameyama M, Imaoka S, *et al.* Increased expression of sialyl Lewisx antigen correlates with poor survival in patients with colorectal carcinoma: clinicopathological and immunohistochemical study. Cancer Res 1993; 53(15): 3632-7.
[PMID: 8101764]

[87]   Nakamori S, Furukawa H, Hiratsuka M, *et al.* Expression of carbohydrate antigen sialyl Le(a): a new functional prognostic factor in gastric cancer. J Clin Oncol 1997; 15(2): 816-25.
[PMID: 9053509]

[88]   Häyry V, Mäkinen LK, Atula T, *et al.* Bmi-1 expression predicts prognosis in squamous cell carcinoma of the tongue. Br J Cancer 2010; 102(5): 892-7.
[PMID: 20145620]

[89]   Ge N, Lin HX, Xiao XS, *et al.* Prognostic significance of Oct4 and Sox2 expression in hypopharyngeal squamous cell carcinoma. J Transl Med 2010; 8: 94.

[PMID: 20937145]

[90] Rietbergen MM, Martens-de Kemp SR, Bloemena E, *et al.* Cancer stem cell enrichment marker CD98: a prognostic factor for survival in patients with human papillomavirus-positive oropharyngeal cancer. Eur J Cancer 2014; 50(4): 765-73.
[PMID: 24315751]

[91] Tanei T, Morimoto K, Shimazu K, *et al.* Association of breast cancer stem cells identified by aldehyde dehydrogenase 1 expression with resistance to sequential Paclitaxel and epirubicin-based chemotherapy for breast cancers. Clin Cancer Res 2009; 15(12): 4234-41.
[PMID: 19509181]

[92] Dan T, Hewitt SM, Ohri N, *et al.* CD44 is prognostic for overall survival in the NCI randomized trial on breast conservation with 25 year follow-up. Breast Cancer Res Treat 2014; 143(1): 11-8.
[PMID: 24276281]

[93] Aomatsu N, Yashiro M, Kashiwagi S, *et al.* CD133 is a useful surrogate marker for predicting chemosensitivity to neoadjuvant chemotherapy in breast cancer. PLoS One 2012; 7(9): e45865.
[PMID: 23049880]

[94] Wang Y, Zhe H, Ding Z, Gao P, Zhang N, Li G. Cancer stem cell marker Bmi-1 expression is associated with basal-like phenotype and poor survival in breast cancer. World J Surg 2012; 36(5): 1189-94.
[PMID: 22366984]

[95] Mylona E, Giannopoulou I, Fasomytakis E, *et al.* The clinicopathologic and prognostic significance of CD44+/CD24(-/low) and CD44-/CD24+ tumor cells in invasive breast carcinomas. Hum Pathol 2008; 39(7): 1096-102.
[PMID: 18495204]

[96] Salnikov AV, Gladkich J, Moldenhauer G, Volm M, Mattern J, Herr I. CD133 is indicative for a resistance phenotype but does not represent a prognostic marker for survival of non-small cell lung cancer patients. Int J Cancer 2010; 126(4): 950-8.
[PMID: 19676044]

[97] Woo T, Okudela K, Mitsui H, *et al.* Prognostic value of CD133 expression in stage I lung adenocarcinomas. Int J Clin Exp Pathol 2010; 4(1): 32-42.
[PMID: 21228926]

[98] Shien K, Toyooka S, Ichimura K, *et al.* Prognostic impact of cancer stem cell-related markers in non-small cell lung cancer patients treated with induction chemoradiotherapy. Lung Cancer 2012; 77(1): 162-7.
[PMID: 22387005]

[99] Ishigami S, Ueno S, Arigami T, *et al.* Prognostic impact of CD133 expression in gastric carcinoma. Anticancer Res 2010; 30(6): 2453-7.
[PMID: 20651407]

[100] Ryu HS, Park DJ, Kim HH, Kim WH, Lee HS. Combination of epithelial-mesenchymal transition and cancer stem cell-like phenotypes has independent prognostic value in gastric cancer. Hum Pathol 2012; 43(4): 520-8.
[PMID: 22018628]

[101] Cao L, Hu X, Zhang J, Liang P, Zhang Y. CD44(+) CD324(-) expression and prognosis in gastric cancer patients. J Surg Oncol 2014; 110(6): 727-33.
[PMID: 24910454]

[102] Yamashita T, Forgues M, Wang W, *et al.* EpCAM and alpha-fetoprotein expression defines novel prognostic subtypes of hepatocellular carcinoma. Cancer Res 2008; 68(5): 1451-61.
[PMID: 18316609]

[103] Song W, Li H, Tao K, *et al.* Expression and clinical significance of the stem cell marker CD133 in hepatocellular carcinoma. Int J Clin Pract 2008; 62(8): 1212-8.
[PMID: 18479363]

[104] Zhao YM, Zhou JM, Wang LR, *et al.* HIWI is associated with prognosis in patients with hepatocellular carcinoma after curative resection. Cancer 2012; 118(10): 2708-17.
[PMID: 21989785]

[105] Guo Z, Li LQ, Jiang JH, Ou C, Zeng LX, Xiang BD. Cancer stem cell markers correlate with early recurrence and survival in hepatocellular carcinoma. World J Gastroenterol 2014; 20(8): 2098-106.
[PMID: 24616575]

[106] Kahlert C, Bergmann F, Beck J, *et al.* Low expression of aldehyde dehydrogenase 1A1 (ALDH1A1) is a prognostic marker for poor survival in pancreatic cancer. BMC Cancer 2011; 11: 275.
[PMID: 21708005]

[107] Ohara Y, Oda T, Sugano M, *et al.* Histological and prognostic importance of CD44(+) /CD24(+) /EpCAM(+) expression in clinical pancreatic cancer. Cancer Sci 2013; 104(8): 1127-34.
[PMID: 23679813]

[108] Hou YC, Chao YJ, Tung HL, Wang HC, Shan YS. Coexpression of CD44-positive/CD133-positive cancer stem cells and CD204-positive tumor-associated macrophages is a predictor of survival in pancreatic ductal adenocarcinoma. Cancer 2014; 120(17): 2766-77.
[PMID: 24839953]

[109] Horst D, Kriegl L, Engel J, Kirchner T, Jung A. CD133 expression is an independent prognostic marker for low survival in colorectal cancer. Br J Cancer 2008; 99(8): 1285-9.
[PMID: 18781171]

[110] Kahlert C, Gaitzsch E, Steinert G, *et al.* Expression analysis of aldehyde dehydrogenase 1A1 (ALDH1A1) in colon and rectal cancer in association with prognosis and response to chemotherapy. Ann Surg Oncol 2012; 19(13): 4193-201.
[PMID: 22878609]

[111] Li T, Su Y, Mei Y, *et al.* ALDH1A1 is a marker for malignant prostate stem cells and predictor of prostate cancer patients' outcome. Lab Invest 2010; 90(2): 234-44.
[PMID: 20010854]

[112] de Resende MF, Chinen LT, Vieira S, *et al.* Prognostication of OCT4 isoform expression in prostate cancer. Tumour Biol 2013; 34(5): 2665-73.
[PMID: 23636800]

[113] Su Y, Qiu Q, Zhang X, *et al.* Aldehyde dehydrogenase 1 A1-positive cell population is enriched in tumor-initiating cells and associated with progression of bladder cancer. Cancer Epidemiol Biomarkers

Prev 2010; 19(2): 327-37.
[PMID: 20142235]

[114] Ferrandina G, Martinelli E, Petrillo M, *et al.* CD133 antigen expression in ovarian cancer. BMC Cancer 2009; 9: 221.
[PMID: 19583859]

[115] Rahadiani N, Ikeda J, Mamat S, *et al.* Expression of aldehyde dehydrogenase 1 (ALDH1) in endometrioid adenocarcinoma and its clinical implications. Cancer Sci 2011; 102(4): 903-8.
[PMID: 21231983]

[116] Meng E, Long B, Sullivan P, *et al.* CD44+/CD24- ovarian cancer cells demonstrate cancer stem cell properties and correlate to survival. Clin Exp Metastasis 2012; 29(8): 939-48.
[PMID: 22610780]

[117] Rot S, Taubert H, Bache M, *et al.* A novel splice variant of the stem cell marker LGR5/GPR49 is correlated with the risk of tumor-related death in soft-tissue sarcoma patients. BMC Cancer 2011; 11: 429.
[PMID: 21978106]

[118] Bleau AM, Agliano A, Larzabal L, de Aberasturi AL, Calvo A. Metastatic dormancy: a complex network between cancer stem cells and their microenvironment. Histol Histopathol 2014; 29(12): 1499-510.
[PMID: 24887025]

[119] Valent P. Emerging stem cell concepts for imatinib-resistant chronic myeloid leukaemia: implications for the biology, management, and therapy of the disease. Br J Haematol 2008; 142(3): 361-78.
[PMID: 18540942]

[120] Singh A, Settleman J. EMT, cancer stem cells and drug resistance: an emerging axis of evil in the war on cancer. Oncogene 2010; 29(34): 4741-51.
[PMID: 20531305]

[121] Schulenburg A, Blatt K, Cerny-Reiterer S, *et al.* Cancer stem cells in basic science and in translational oncology: can we translate into clinical application? J Hematol Oncol 2015; 8(1): 16.
[PMID: 25886184]

[122] Carrasco E, Alvarez PJ, Prados J, *et al.* Cancer stem cells and their implication in breast cancer. Eur J Clin Invest 2014; 44(7): 678-87.
[PMID: 24766664]

[123] Zhang W, Lei P, Dong X, Xu C. The new concepts on overcoming drug resistance in lung cancer. Drug Des Devel Ther 2014; 8: 735-44.
[PMID: 24944510]

[124] Findlay VJ, Wang C, Watson DK, Camp ER. Epithelial-to-mesenchymal transition and the cancer stem cell phenotype: insights from cancer biology with therapeutic implications for colorectal cancer. Cancer Gene Ther 2014; 21(5): 181-7.
[PMID: 24787239]

[125] Guddati AK. Ovarian cancer stem cells: elusive targets for chemotherapy. Med Oncol 2012; 29(5): 3400-8.

[PMID: 22638913]

[126] Ischenko I, Seeliger H, Jauch KW, Bruns CJ. Metastatic activity and chemotherapy resistance in human pancreatic cancer--influence of cancer stem cells. Surgery 2009; 146(3): 430-4.
[PMID: 19715799]

[127] Sekulic A, Migden MR, Oro AE, *et al.* Efficacy and safety of vismodegib in advanced basal-cell carcinoma. N Engl J Med 2012; 366(23): 2171-9.
[PMID: 22670903]

[128] Chapman PB, Hauschild A, Robert C, *et al.* Improved survival with vemurafenib in melanoma with BRAF V600E mutation. N Engl J Med 2011; 364(26): 2507-16.
[PMID: 21639808]

[129] Galanis E, Buckner JC, Maurer MJ, *et al.* Phase II trial of temsirolimus (CCI-779) in recurrent glioblastoma multiforme: a North Central Cancer Treatment Group Study. J Clin Oncol 2005; 23(23): 5294-304.
[PMID: 15998902]

[130] Hudes GR. mTOR as a target for therapy of renal cancer. Clin Adv Hematol Oncol 2007; 5(10): 772-4.
[PMID: 17998894]

[131] Moore MJ, Goldstein D, Hamm J, *et al.* Erlotinib plus gemcitabine compared with gemcitabine alone in patients with advanced pancreatic cancer: a phase III trial of the National Cancer Institute of Canada Clinical Trials Group. J Clin Oncol 2007; 25(15): 1960-6.
[PMID: 17452677]

[132] Geyer CE, Forster J, Lindquist D, *et al.* Lapatinib plus capecitabine for HER2-positive advanced breast cancer. N Engl J Med 2006; 355(26): 2733-43.
[PMID: 17192538]

[133] Blay JY, Le Cesne A, Ray-Coquard I, *et al.* Prospective multicentric randomized phase III study of imatinib in patients with advanced gastrointestinal stromal tumors comparing interruption *versus* continuation of treatment beyond 1 year: the French Sarcoma Group. J Clin Oncol 2007; 25(9): 1107-13.
[PMID: 17369574]

[134] Cunningham D, Humblet Y, Siena S, *et al.* Cetuximab monotherapy and cetuximab plus irinotecan in irinotecan-refractory metastatic colorectal cancer. N Engl J Med 2004; 351(4): 337-45.
[PMID: 15269313]

[135] Jonker DJ, O'Callaghan CJ, Karapetis CS, *et al.* Cetuximab for the treatment of colorectal cancer. N Engl J Med 2007; 357(20): 2040-8.
[PMID: 18003960]

[136] Vogel CL, Cobleigh MA, Tripathy D, *et al.* Efficacy and safety of trastuzumab as a single agent in first-line treatment of HER2-overexpressing metastatic breast cancer. J Clin Oncol 2002; 20(3): 719-26.
[PMID: 11821453]

[137] Swain SM, Baselga J, Kim SB, *et al.* Pertuzumab, trastuzumab, and docetaxel in HER2-positive metastatic breast cancer. N Engl J Med 2015; 372(8): 724-34.

[PMID: 25693012]

[138] Bang YJ, Van Cutsem E, Feyereislova A, *et al.* Trastuzumab in combination with chemotherapy versus chemotherapy alone for treatment of HER2-positive advanced gastric or gastro-oesophageal junction cancer (ToGA): a phase 3, open-label, randomised controlled trial. Lancet 2010; 376(9742): 687-97.
[PMID: 20728210]

[139] Bookman MA, Darcy KM, Clarke-Pearson D, Boothby RA, Horowitz IR. Evaluation of monoclonal humanized anti-HER2 antibody, trastuzumab, in patients with recurrent or refractory ovarian or primary peritoneal carcinoma with overexpression of HER2: a phase II trial of the Gynecologic Oncology Group. J Clin Oncol 2003; 21(2): 283-90.
[PMID: 12525520]

[140] Perez EA, Romond EH, Suman VJ, *et al.* Trastuzumab plus adjuvant chemotherapy for human epidermal growth factor receptor 2-positive breast cancer: planned joint analysis of overall survival from NSABP B-31 and NCCTG N9831. J Clin Oncol 2014; 32(33): 3744-52.
[PMID: 25332249]

[141] Tolaney SM, Barry WT, Dang CT, *et al.* Adjuvant paclitaxel and trastuzumab for node-negative, HER2-positive breast cancer. N Engl J Med 2015; 372(2): 134-41.
[PMID: 25564897]

[142] Herrmann H, Sadovnik I, Cerny-Reiterer S, *et al.* Dipeptidylpeptidase IV (CD26) defines leukemic stem cells (LSC) in chronic myeloid leukemia. Blood 2014; 123(25): 3951-62.
[PMID: 24778155]

[143] de Gramont A, Tournigand C, André T, Larsen AK, Louvet C. Targeted agents for adjuvant therapy of colon cancer. Semin Oncol 2006; 33(6) (Suppl. 11): S42-5.
[PMID: 17178286]

[144] Cohen DJ, Hochster HS. Update on clinical data with regimens inhibiting angiogenesis and epidermal growth factor receptor for patients with newly diagnosed metastatic colorectal cancer. Clin Colorectal Cancer 2007; 7 (Suppl. 1): S21-7.
[PMID: 18361803]

[145] Al-Husein B, Abdalla M, Trepte M, Deremer DL, Somanath PR. Antiangiogenic therapy for cancer: an update. Pharmacotherapy 2012; 32(12): 1095-111.
[PMID: 23208836]

[146] Van Loon K, Venook AP. Adjuvant treatment of colon cancer: what is next? Curr Opin Oncol 2011; 23(4): 403-9.
[PMID: 21537178]

[147] Allegra CJ, Yothers G, O'Connell MJ, *et al.* Phase III trial assessing bevacizumab in stages II and III carcinoma of the colon: results of NSABP protocol C-08. J Clin Oncol 2011; 29(1): 11-6.
[PMID: 20940184]

[148] Oyan B. Why do targeted agents not work in the adjuvant setting in colon cancer? Expert Rev Anticancer Ther 2012; 12(10): 1337-45.
[PMID: 23176621]

[149] Mountzios G, Pentheroudakis G, Carmeliet P. Bevacizumab and micrometastases: revisiting the preclinical and clinical rollercoaster. Pharmacol Ther 2014; 141(2): 117-24.
[PMID: 24076268]

[150] Gandhi S, Fletcher GG, Eisen A, *et al.* Adjuvant chemotherapy for early female breast cancer: a systematic review of the evidence for the 2014 Cancer Care Ontario systemic therapy guideline. Curr Oncol 2015; 22 (Suppl. 1): S82-94.
[PMID: 25848343]

SUBJECT INDEX